THE COLIBAN MAIN CHANNEL
A Walking Guide

Stephen Charman

THE COLIBAN MAIN CHANNEL – A Walking Guide

Copyright © Stephen Charman, 2023

All rights reserved. Without limiting the rights under copyright, no part of this publication may be reproduced, stored or introduced into a retrieval system, or transmitted in any form or by any means (electronic, mechanical, photocopying, recording or otherwise) without the prior written permission of the writer and the publisher.

ISBN: 978 0 6486574 4 6

All historic photos have been obtained from the State Library website unless otherwise indicated.

While the author and publisher have made every reasonable effort to locate, contact and acknowledge copyright owners, any copyright owners who are not properly identified and acknowledged should contact the publisher so that corrections can be made in the next edition

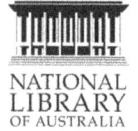 A catalogue record for this book is available from the National Library of Australia

Harcourt Heritage & Tourist Centre

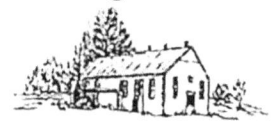

Contents

The Author	v
Acknowledgements	vii
Introduction	1
History of The Coliban Water Scheme	5
Walking the Coliban Water Scheme	10
Malmsbury Reservoir to Forrest Road	13
The Back Creek Syphon	37
The Failure of the First Back Creek Syphon	42
Back Creek Syphon Outlet to Taradale Road	47
Taradale Road to Fryerstown Road	52
Fryerstown Road to Wright Street, Elphinstone	60
Wright Street, Elphinstone to Elphinstone township	64
The Channel at Elphinstone	68
Elphinstone to Ellerys Road, Faraday	74
Porters Tunnel to Expedition Pass Reservoir	84
Ellerys Road, Faraday to Faraday-Sutton Grange Road	94
Faraday-Sutton Grange Road to Harcourt-Sutton Grange Road	105
Harcourt-Sutton Grange Road to Youngs Lane, Harcourt North	126
Youngs Lane, Harcourt North to Blossett Drive, Mandurang South	132
Blossett Drive to Harpers Road	151
Harpers Road to Sandhurst Reservoir	160
Sandhurst Reservoir to No. 7 Reservoir	172
The Three Reservoirs Circuit Walk	184
No. 7 Reservoir to Kangaroo Flat Railway Station	207
Epilogue	211
Glossary	212

The Author

Stephen is a keen bushwalker and naturalist with a love of local history, as well as having a long history in community radio. Stephen's music show 'Open Tuning' has been on the air on Castlemaine's 94.9 MainFM for fourteen years. Before this he did radio programs on PhoenixFM Bendigo, and RRRFM and PBSFM in Melbourne.

Stephen lives just a short stroll from the Coliban Main Channel, not far from the '18 mile post', the point where the Main Channel diverges from the now decommissioned Harcourt and Expedition Pass Reservoir Channels.

Note:

Throughout the book, wherever there is an excerpt from a newspaper, spellings have been kept as they were in the original article. Outside of the excerpts, the more conventional spelling of place names, in particular, is used. For example, in the original article, mention is made of Porter's Tunnel. The caption to the accompanying photo has Porters Tunnel.

Acknowledgements

My thanks to members of the Friends of Wattle Gully and Chewton Facebook group, in particular, Lani Smith who posted on the group's page a photo she labelled: 'Castlemaine District, Victoria, ca 1894. People standing on the water race at Whisky Gully near Mount Alexander [eastern side], creator: M. Law (photographer). (Museums Victoria)' (see page 115). This photo sent me off to find the precise locations of a raft of historic photos of the Coliban Main Channel that, through her encouragement, I found on the State Library Victoria website.

The help of the Harcourt Heritage Centre for auspicing this project is most appreciated. In particular I'd like to thank George Milford for his advice and encouragement and Bernie Schultz for taking on the onerous task of proofreading, copy editing and book layout. And to Jase Haysom for suggesting I visit the Harcourt Heritage Centre in the first place.

And thanks to Rod Andrew, retired engineer with the State Rivers and Water Supply Commission, who lent me some key reference texts and helped me fix some early errors.

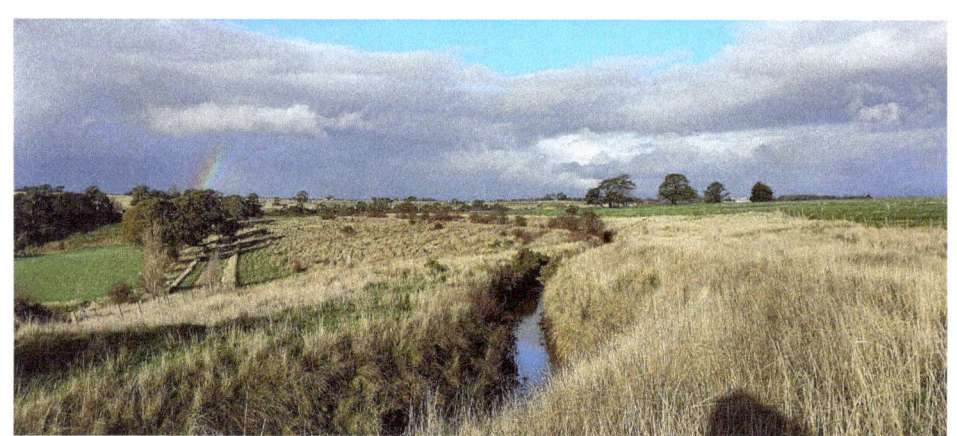

Coliban Main Channel, Malmsbury.

Introduction

In November 1877 water finally began to flow from Malmsbury Reservoir to Crusoe Reservoir Bendigo signalling the end of the first construction phase of the complete Coliban Water Scheme and the beginning of a reliable water supply for Bendigo. In 2022, my love of history and bushwalking led me to examine the Coliban Main Channel in detail. It wasn't long before a search of Trove led me to a series of newspaper articles written by unnamed reporters, the majority writing before 1900, which gave some context for the historical relics I was noticing as I walked the length of the Main Channel. I took a special interest in visiting sites that had been photographed, sometimes a hundred and fifty years before (most sourced from the State Library website). My aim was to take photographs that matched (wherever possible) the original view. The result was this book, which combines those photographs with selections from the early articles written as the Coliban Water Scheme neared completion.

In this second edition, I have taken the opportunity to incorporate a more detailed description of the channel, including suggested walks and maps. This has entailed dividing the Channel into sections more suitable for walkers who would like a variety of walk suggestions, both long and short.

A number of contemporary writers have written about the Coliban Water Scheme. I thank Rod Andrew, a retired SR&WSC water engineer for giving me an electronic copy of his own study on the Coliban Main Channel, prepared for the Malmsbury Historical Society. His book *Malmsbury reservoir: A history in news articles and pictures* (self published, 2014) is an insightful and detailed look at the troubled history of the construction of the Malmsbury Reservoir. Some of this information is also contained in Geoffrey Russell's *Water For Gold: The Fight to Quench Central Victoria's Goldfields* (2009), the story behind the creation of the Coliban Water Scheme and, while now out of print, is readily available at most public libraries. Through Rod I was also able to obtain a copy of Philip Wilkin's *Along the Channel: Some of the historical and general features along the Coliban Main Channel* (self published, 2012) which describes Philip's own observations as he rode and walked the Main Channel in 2011 and 2012. While I wasn't aware of Philip Wilkin's book when I started putting this book together (at the time, Philip's limited edition book was out of print),[1] the similarities are striking and remind us that if you think you've got a good idea you can pretty well bet someone else has had the same idea before you.

At any rate, both Philip's book and this one come out of a love for history, as well as the sheer pleasure to be had from rambling and exploring. Hopefully, both studies will inspire people to get out and see for themselves the historical and scenic features of the Coliban Main Channel. There are certainly challenges for the keen walker who decides to tackle the complete walk. Some sections aren't readily accessible, others might be accessible but aren't maintained, and there are all sorts of obstacles to be surmounted, including locked gates, errant cattle, and, as I discovered, a good number of snakes hiding in the long grass. The walker needs to be prepared for the occasional detour before the channel access track can be rejoined. Still, what's life without a few challenges? Over a couple of weeks in late 2022 I did indeed manage to walk pretty much the complete channel system. My aim was not only to see what remained of the original 1870s channel, these days much altered, but also to build up a picture of how the original channel might have looked. Given the phenomenal amount of rain that fell during the spring of 2022, the prolific growth of grass and weeds, and the subsequent damage done to access tracks, the challenge was even greater than normal!

The Coliban Main Channel remains a fascinating and, perhaps, under-appreciated regional attraction which provides plenty of scope for sightseeing and hiking. It is to be hoped that one day a trail might be constructed that allows walkers to travel the length of the Main Channel, possibly dovetailing with the Leanganook Track to allow a choice of paths and the opportunity to create a different return route for hikers wanting to circle back to their starting point.

---

1 Philip Wilkin's book can be printed on request by the Malmsbury Historical Society. A copy is available from the National Library of Australia.

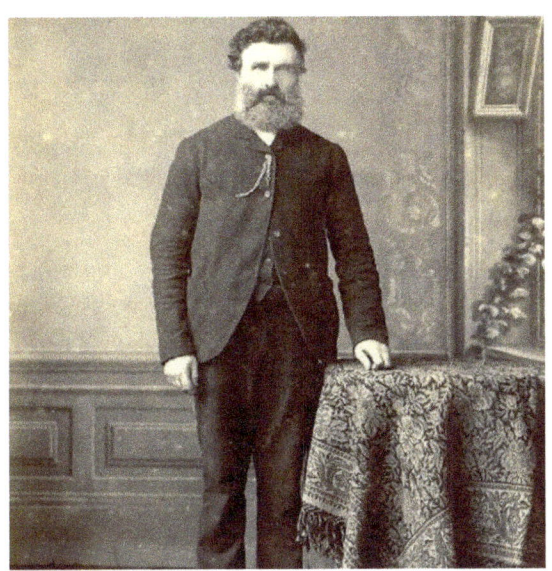

Joseph Brady, Chief Engineer, Coliban Water Scheme.

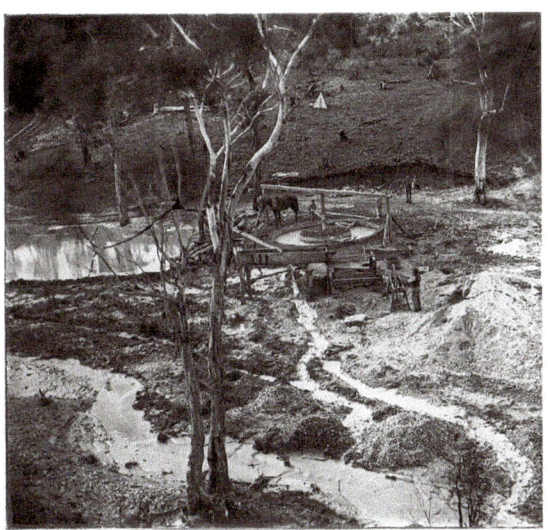

An example of a horse-powered puddling machine.

History of The Coliban Water Scheme

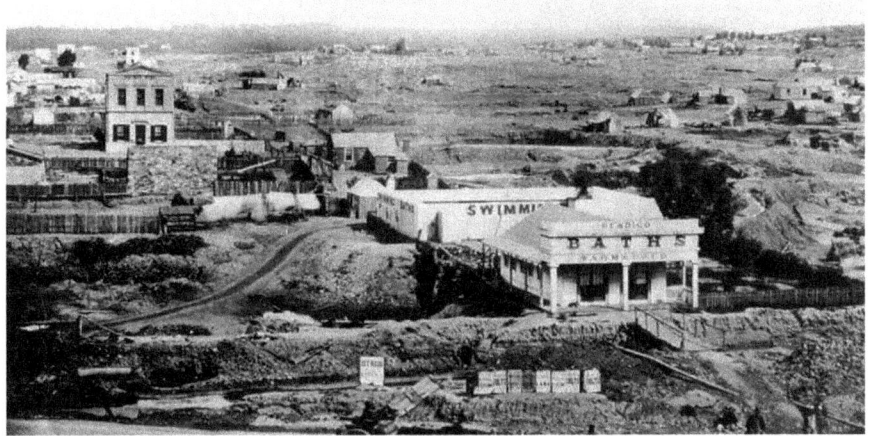

Sandhurst (Bendigo) in the 1850s.

The discovery of gold in Central Victoria in 1861 resulted in an influx of fossickers eager to try their luck and, hopefully, make their fortunes. The rich Castlemaine and Bendigo goldfields attracted the largest congregation of diggers and their families in those early years. Very quickly, tent cities sprang up, placing great pressure on the existing water resources of the area. Not only did the new arrivals need water for their personal use, gold mining was an extremely thirsty industry. It soon became obvious that for the new towns and industries to remain viable, the Government had to step in and find sufficient water for their needs.

> 'As far back as 1860, if not earlier, general attention was directed to the scarcity of water in the Castlemaine and Sandhurst districts, and various schemes were suggested whereby the deficiency could be supplied. At Sandhurst[2] in times of drought the rates charged for water rose to famine

---

2 Sandhurst changed its name to Bendigo on 8 May 1891. It will be assumed that the reader knows that both names refer to the same locality.

prices, and the almost absurd sums paid for buckets of water not unnaturally gave rise to sanguine speculations as to the profits that were in store for the company that would bring in a copious supply of water to the rich goldfields of Castlemaine and Sandhurst. It frequently happened that when there was a drought at Sandhurst, the Coliban and Campaspe rivers overflowed their banks, and on one occasion one of those casual observations that sometimes give rise to great schemes was dropped. It is stated that a gentleman resident at Sandhurst said to a friend of his, a resident of the Coliban district, "What a pity it is you cannot give us some of your floods, and you take some of our dry weather in exchange" … The idea was started, and it is likely it was started in some such way, for the ever pressing necessities of Castlemaine and Sandhurst would naturally give rise to the invention.

Like all costly schemes the proposal enlisted the sympathies of several enthusiasts. No fewer than three rival schemes were soon propounded, three surveys and sections were made, and the Government were asked to concede water rights and privileges with the view of forming a company to carry out the undertaking. A Parliamentary committee was appointed on the 9th December 1864 to inquire into the project, examine the rival surveys, and advise the Government generally on the subject. The report of this committee, prepared on the 18th May 1865, first gave the present scheme tangible form and direction.

The three schemes mentioned above were propounded by Mr. [Edward] Wardle, Mr. [Joseph] Brady and Mr. [John] Reilly. The committee reported that neither of the schemes as submitted contained within itself the general principles which they regarded as essential, and that they considered those principles would be best attained by an amalgamation of portions of the schemes of Mr. Brady and Mr. Wardle. The committee also recommended the constructions of the upper and lower reservoirs on the Coliban, though up to the present time [1878] only the lower one has been built, viz., that in view of the railway station at Malmsbury.

Of the two lines of aqueduct, the committee most strongly commended that proposed by Mr. Brady as the shortest and best, and that Mr. Wardle should receive full consideration

from the Government for the valuable scheme put forward by him. They also recommended that the supply should be carried out by the State, and not by private enterprise. The report of the committee was adopted, and the undertaking was commenced on the 1st June 1866, under Mr. Christopherson as chief engineer, Mr. Shakespeare being appointed resident engineer at Malmsbury, and Mr. Mouline resident engineer at Sandhurst.'
The Age, January 2 1878, p. 2.

Before the construction of the Coliban Water Scheme, the Irish engineer Joseph Brady had devised a plan to create eight reservoirs along the Bendigo valley, six for mining purposes and two for domestic purposes.[3] Some of these reservoirs still exist. No. 7 Reservoir at Big Hill, as it's name implies, was one of the proposed series. This reservoir, as well as Crusoe Reservoir (built in 1873), both now decommissioned, provided much needed water supplies for Sandhurst, but the catchments of both these reservoirs were of insufficient size to ensure water security. The present day Sandhurst Reservoir is close to the proposed location of No. 8 Reservoir.

The three schemes considered by the committee were all broadly similar. Each recommended the excavation of an aqueduct or channel connecting a reservoir to be built near Malmsbury to

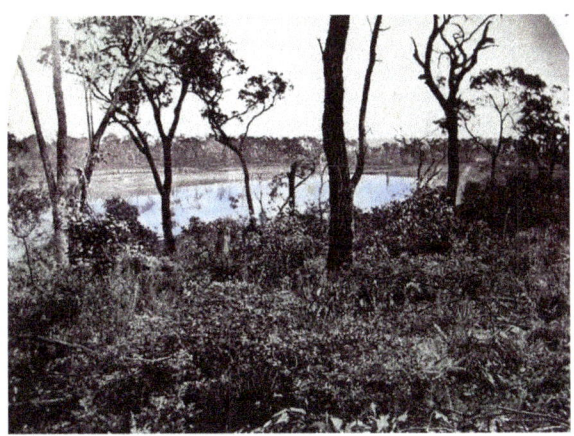

Reservoir No. 1, Golden Square, 1861.

---

3   *Joseph Brady's Coliban System of Waterworks*, Coliban Water pamphlet.

No. 7 Reservoir at Big Hill. This entailed the construction of a series of tunnels beneath intervening ridges, at least two syphons (buried pipes) spanning creek valleys, and numerous flumes (elevated timber and brick 'bridges') to carry water across gullies and depressions. While the three proposals were broadly similar, John Reilly's scheme would have meant a more elevated channel, requiring a more tortuous course. For instance, to take the water from Malmsbury Reservoir to Elphinstone, Joseph Brady's scheme would lead to a race 26 km in length, Reilly's channel would have been 69 km long, and the channel designed by the other applicant, Edward Wardle, would have been 44 km.[4]

Before a decision was made, Wardle and Reilly battled on behalf of their schemes.

> 'Mr. Wardle then entered upon a lengthy and detailed explanation of how at one point Mr. Reilly's race ran twenty feet below his own, and at another point 160 feet above. These were both points below the starting-point and the fact was irreconcilable with a correct level.'
> *The Argus Wednesday 16 November 1864, p. 6.*

Joseph Brady's scheme had also gained favour by allowing a generous allocation of compensation water to landowners along the banks of the Coliban, whereas the other applicants hadn't considered this question. Brady also seemed to have had a more realistic estimation of the amount of water that could be farmed and sent down the channel.

However, once the project began it soon ran into problems. By 1869 the State Government's Engineer-in-Chief, Thomas Higinbotham, was raising serious doubts about how the project was progressing. His concerns, outlined in the *Bendigo Advertiser* 13 February of that year, included the ballooning cost of the project due to blatant rorting by some of the project's contractors and, more worryingly, the deficiencies in the construction of Malmsbury Reservoir, especially the poorly designed and constructed outlet which ran through the embankment wall. In particular, he bemoaned the oversight in letting the contract for the construction of the dam without including in it the cost of the

---

4   *Bendigo Advertiser*, 27 February 1865, p. 3 (Mr. Christopherson's Report).

outlet works and water tower, the erection of which was necessary before the embankment could be completed. His fears were borne out soon enough. The following year Christopherson's recklessness and incompetence would put the whole Coliban Water Scheme in peril. It not only led to the dramatic failure of the Back Creek syphon, integral to the success of the scheme, but it would lead to, what seemed at the time, the near collapse of the Malmsbury reservoir. Needless to say, this latter event caused a sensation in the township of Malmsbury which lay just below the reservoir.

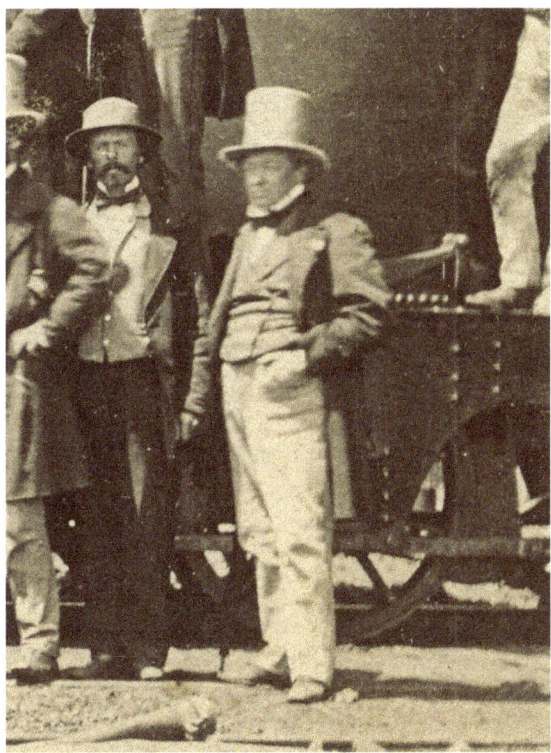

Coliban Water Scheme: The first Chief Engineer, Henry Christopherson (centre).

Walking the Coliban Water Scheme

It seems rather obvious to say that the best way to get to know the Coliban Main Channel is by exploring it, either in part or in total. However the latter is not an easy task, or even possible, as some sections are inaccessible, some are within freehold land, and as the Channel is still in operation, sections may be closed off for maintenance from time to time.

Nevertheless, throughout the book maps have been provided which offer suggestions for walkers keen to see some (or most) of the channel. While the access tracks are well maintained and marked along some stretches of the channel, in other parts, they are indiscernible or non-existent. The average walker might be wise to skip those sections. However, for the sake of completeness, I've included a description of those parts of the channel that the majority of walkers won't wish to explore, or are unable to access.

The first edition of this book revolved around newspaper articles[5] which contained descriptions of the channel around the time it was constructed in the 1870s. In addition, historic photos were provided to help walkers visualise how notable features of the channel might once have appeared. For the most part these historic articles and photos have been retained but are now augmented by walking notes and maps. Each section walk is of greater or lesser length and difficulty.

Is it possible to walk the entire channel with a couple of overnight stops? Unfortunately, not yet, unless you're happy to trudge kilometres along the shoulders of some very narrow and dangerous secondary roads. Not only wouldn't I recommend this, I would advise against it given the danger of a driver failing to see walkers on the road. Nevertheless, it's quite possible to walk a large part of the channel with an overnight stay either at the Leanganook camping area within the Mount Alexander Regional Park or at the Goom Gooruduron-yeran Campground at Mandurang South. The latter, at the time of writing, doesn't have toilets. In addition, clean drinking water may or may not be available at both these locations, depending on demand and time of year.

---

5   Newspaper articles have been sourced from trove.nla.gov.au

'...It will not come within the scope of these papers to enter into a political history of the Coliban Scheme, but rather to state what it was originally intended to be, what it is now expected it will be, and, above all, to endeavor[6] to thoroughly acquaint the public with the present condition of the works from the Malmsbury channel to the last pipe in Eaglehawk.[7] In entering upon the task- i.e. upon the examination of the works ... I have arrived at the conclusion that the best plan is to take readers with me over the works, step by step and to do my "level best" to make them see with their mind's eye what I saw with my bodily eyes, leaving them as much as possible to draw their own deductions.

> **COMPLETION OF THE SANDHURST SECTION OF THE COLIBAN WATER SUPPLY SCHEME.**
>
> [BY OUR SPECIAL REPORTER.]
>
> The completion of the last portion of the "Coliban Scheme" is now an accomplished fact, but there are numbers of persons in Sandhurst who still look upon it as a myth, and will not be convinced of its practical character until the water is actually running into the Crusoe Gully Reservoir, which, however, barring accidents, it *will* do within a very few days. On receiving my instructions I proceeded to Castlemaine and inspected the works from the Expedition Pass Reservoir, along the channel leading into it to the point of divergence of the Sandhurst branch at the old 18 mile peg, and from thence to the Crusoe Gully Reservoir. Having a few hours to spare I also went over the principal sluicing claims, some account of which I will give in another paper, the particulars of which will, I think, be interesting to those who are anxiously waiting for a supply of water at cheap rates to work the White Hills and other localities.

Extract from The Bendigo Advertiser, November 20, 1877.

---

6 Spellings today that are thought of as American, such as 'color' and 'center', were used globally well into the 20th century. Hence, we have the Australian Labor (not Labour) Party, a reminder of a time before codification took place.

7 This book is primarily concerned with the channel from Malmsbury Reservoir to Crusoe Reservoir..

... Although technical terms will be avoided as much as possible, there are a few which cannot be rid of, and as these will be constantly occurring it may be well as at once to explain them. ... The word "channel" will be used in speaking of the open cuttings in which the water is to be conveyed from reservoir to reservoir, in preference to the word "aqueduct",[8] which, technically speaking, has so often been wrongly applied. ... The "bank" of the channel is simply the ground on either side. ... A "flume" is a construction of stone, brick, wood, or iron, or of combinations of these materials, as the case may be, carrying the water across depressions in the ground, these depressions being either the beds of creeks, dry gullies or caused by subsidence of the soil. A "culvert" is a short tunnel, conveying the water under roadways and railway embankments. With these explanations of the most frequently recurring technicalities and explaining others as they arise, the general reader will, I think, find no difficulty in forming an accurate conception of the character of the works.' [Refer to the Glossary, page 212, for definitions of other terms used in the text.]
The Bendigo Advertiser, January 26 1874, p. 2.

---

8   Nevertheless, some reporters of that time preferred to use the term 'aqueduct' rather than 'channel' in their reports.

Malmsbury Reservoir to Forrest Road

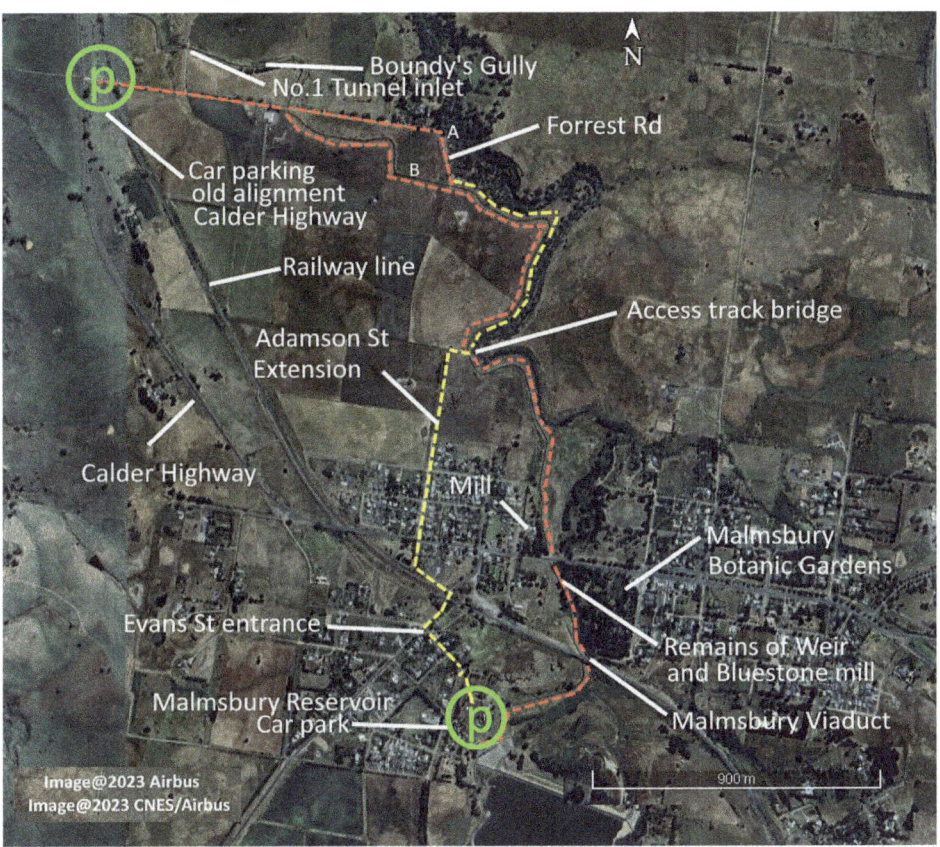

'Everyone who has travelled on the Melbourne and Sandhurst line of railway must, as the train stopped at the prettily situated Malmsbury station, have observed about a quarter of a mile [400 m][9] to the left (if coming up the line) the magnificent embankment which dams the pure waters of the Coliban. The long level stretch of high earthwork, behind which a glimpse is caught of an expanse of blue water hemmed in by hills; the geometrical sweep of the bye-washes at either end; and the

---

9   Metric equivalents are given in square brackets only where it is important for comprehension.

pinnacle of the huge iron tower,[10] whose foundations are buried fathoms deep beneath the surface, together form a picture at once striking and beautiful.'
Bendigo Advertiser, Tuesday 27 January 1874, p. 2.

'Within 50 yards [46 m] of the western angle, formed by the embankment, stands the iron water-tower, which regulates the outflow to the main channel. Most of the party took advantage of the boat, and rowed across to it, and were soon busy exploring the interior. Some even descended to the lowest point above the surface, where the water rushes through the valves with an incessant thunder. On one occasion an adventurous dog fell down the stairway into the swirling mass below when the water was rushing through at the rate of 180 cubic feet per second. Strange to say, he was caught fairly in the current, and whirling through the valves in a second, came out on the embankment wagging his tail. None of the party cared to try and emulate the canine action, and probably they would not have been so fortunate, owing to recent alterations.'
The Sydney Morning Herald, Monday 1 February 1886, p. 6.

'At the Malmsbury reservoir one of the most prominent features is a cemetery situated on elevated ground close to the water's edge. At first sight the danger [of water pollution] from this source appears greater than it really is, for between the burial ground and the water there is a considerable thickness of rock, the strata of which slope away from the reservoir, as also does the general surface of the ground. It cannot, however, be considered that there is no danger at all, for the joints of the rocks— which are at right angles to the place of stratification — slope towards the reservoir, as also does the southern corner of the surface. Another objectionable feature here is that the grazing area extends into the valley of the reservoir on both sides and not only so, but the fence along the water's edge has gaps purposely left in it at intervals to admit of cattle going down to the water to drink. In one place we saw a slip panel in the fence, through which evidently cattle were occasionally

---

10 The original iron outlet tower was demolished and replaced by the current outlet tower in 1900. Rod Andrew, *Malmsbury Reservoir: A history in news articles and pictures*, 2014, p. 37.

admitted to graze ; on one occasion we found a beast grazing there, which on our approach went up to the slip panel to be let out.'
Mt Alexander Mail, Saturday 29 May 1897, p. 2.

The contract for the construction of the Malmsbury Reservoir was let in June 1866 with the completion date August of the following year, but from the start there were problems. Besides the issues previously mentioned, there was considerable friction between Christopherson and the contractor Greenwood which culminated in the sacking of both men. The appointment of a new contractor in 1869 didn't improve matters. Matters came to a head in 1870 when key decisions made earlier proved disastrous. One of these was the importation from England and erection of an insufficiently strong water tower. This meant that the outlet valves regulated by the tower never functioned properly and had to be modified to allow water to flow at a satisfactory rate through an outlet pipe which ran through the embankment wall.[11] But the main problem was the unsuitability of the outlet pipe itself. Christopherson had bought a stock of obsolete Melbourne Sewer Company cast-iron segments which, according to Christopherson's plan, were to be bolted together to form pipes able to be used at both Malmsbury reservoir and the Back Creek syphon.

A journalist in an 1886 report takes up the story:

> 'It is this piece of work which brought the Coliban scheme so unpleasantly prominent before the public some years ago. The mouth of the outlet originally consisted of a cast-iron pipe having an internal diameter of 7 feet 8 inches, which ran between the tower and the embankment, and discharged the water into the open masonry channel. It seems that this, the first pipe laid down here, was never intended for such purpose ; it was too large and weak. Consequently it broke, and gradually became fractured for a distance of nearly 100 feet, and the water instead of going along it poured through the fractures, and threatened to make a clean sweep of the embankment. The void spaces above and around the pipe should have been

---

11 Andrew, p. 48.

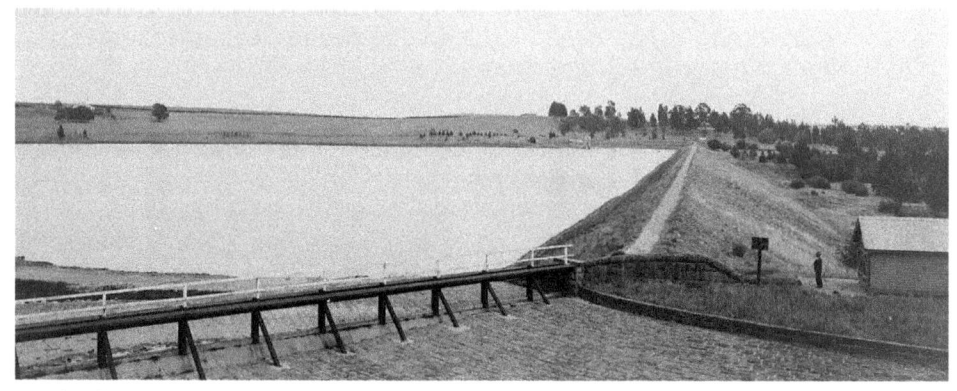
Malmsbury Reservoir, prior to 1939.

filled with puddle, but this not having been done, the waters of course had free play. When the fractures were discovered, Mr. John Woods, late Minister for Railways, and at present a member of Parliament, being then engineer in charge of the works, tarred over all the fractures, though he subsequently stated he did so at the request of his superior officer.

Unfortunately, the ingenious device did not answer. Subsequently, the whole of the fractured pipe was removed by means of a shaft which was sunk through the puddle-wall, and replaced by a brick culvert laid upon a foundation of cement concrete. It was during this operation that the spaces which should have been filled with puddle[12] were found to contain nothing but staves of cement casks, broken bottles, straw, and all sorts of rubbish. Altogether it proved to be one of the prettiest pieces of Government contracting ever brought to light.'
The Sydney Morning Herald, Monday 1 February 1886, p. 6.

After an investigation by an engineer brought over from India, Lieutenant Colonel RH Sankey, the necessary repairs were made and Malmsbury Reservoir was finally completed in 1874. Over time, further improvements have occurred and comparing the early photo of the Reservoir with a contemporary photo (page 18) shows that the old tower was finally replaced and flood control

---

12 Puddle is worked clay which is impervious to water.

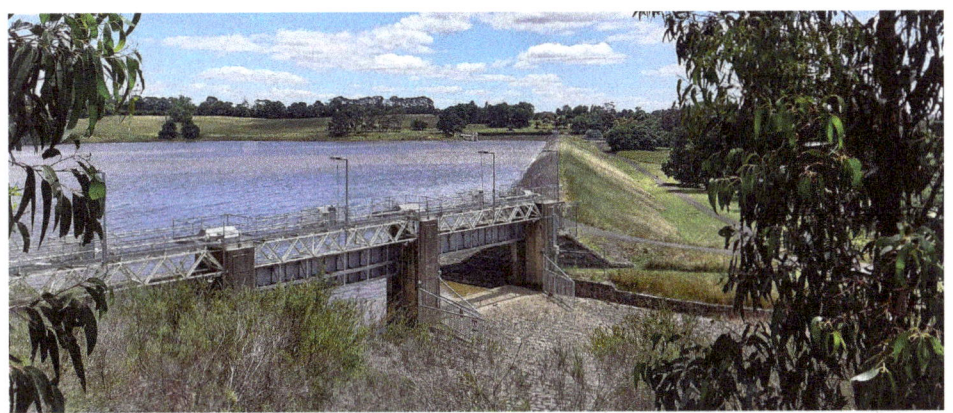

Present day view of previous photo showing increase in height of embankment.

gates on the eastern and western bye-wash installed, the result of which has been the increased capacity of the reservoir.[13]

Today the reservoir is a beautifully maintained and popular tourist destination. It boasts manicured lawns, picnic facilities, a playground and a shelter. It is here, at the Malmsbury Reservoir car park, that any attempt to walk the entire channel must start.

This part of the channel can be explored either as a return walk of 6 km or as a one-way walk if a car shuttle can be organised. Walkers who have parked at the Malmsbury Reservoir car park can choose to return the way they came, or else cross over the channel at Forrest Road and return along a walking track (yellow dashed line) that runs between the channel and the Coliban River.

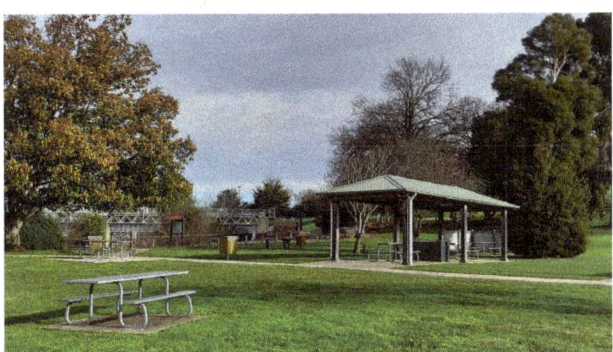

Malmsbury Reservoir Picnic Area.

---

13 The capacity of Malmsbury Reservoir was increased in 1939 by installing flood gates and raising the height of the embankment. Andrew, p. 74.

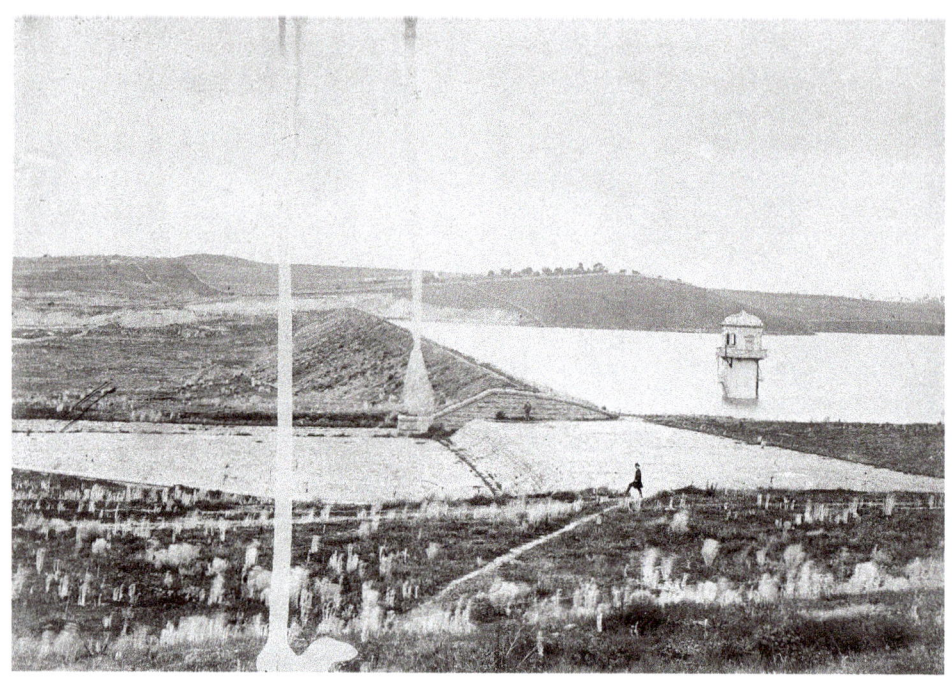

Malmsbury Reservoir showing old tower, 1870s.

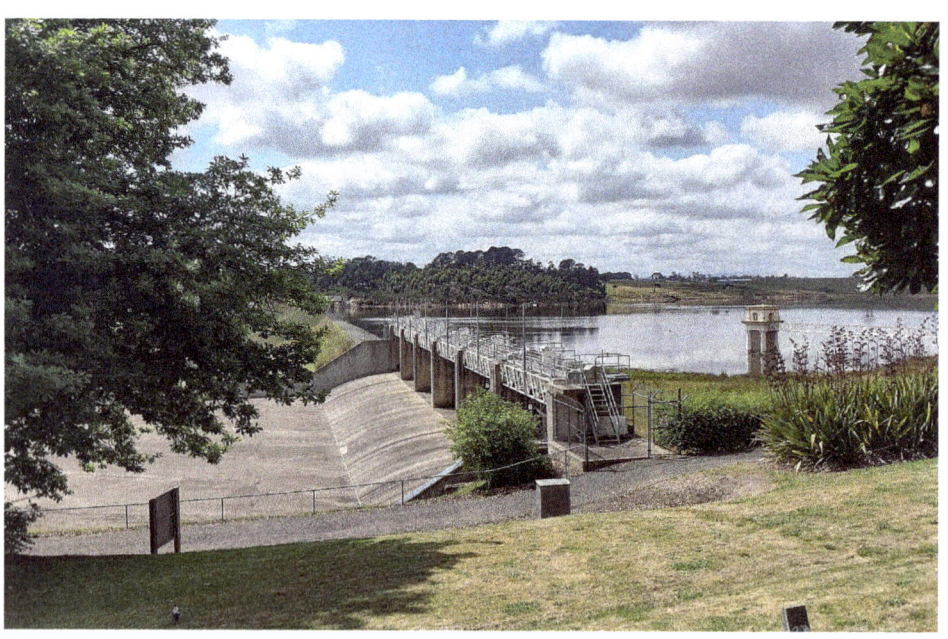

Present day view showing the later tower on the right.

The channel can then be crossed again at the access track bridge and walkers can return to the Reservoir car park along a right of way (Adamson Street extension) and then via Fleming Street and the Daylesford-Malmsbury Road before reaching the car park via the Evans Street, Malmsbury Reservoir entrance.

Walkers who have organised a car shuttle (there is a parking area near the corner of Forrest Road and the Calder Highway at an abandoned alignment of the highway) can either follow the channel within the Coliban water reserve to Forrest Road near Boundy's Gully or by walking the length of Forrest Road.

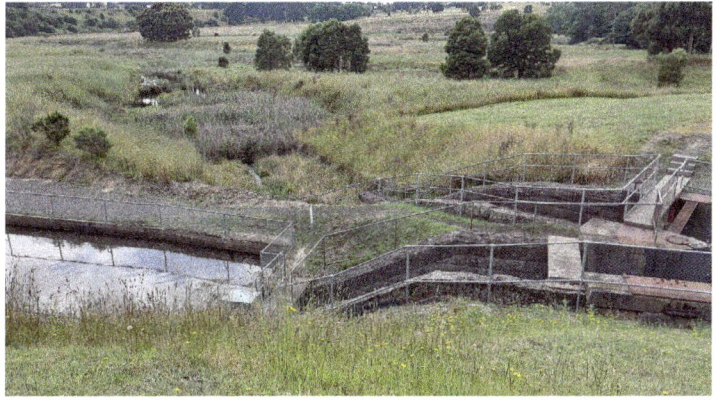

Sluice gates: Main Channel, left foreground. In the middle distance is the compensation channel leading to the Coliban River.

'We now come to the "channel" proper, by which term is designated the open cutting stretching from Malmsbury to Sandhurst, a distance of between forty and fifty miles [64 to 80 km], with its culverts, tunnels, flumes, and weirs, &c., adapting the contour of the ground it passes over to the conveyance of the Coliban Water. ... It is this ground that I hope to get over in the present paper, taking the reader with me along the bank of the channel towards Castlemaine, and will explain objects of interest as we pass them. ... The reader will start with me from the sluice gates, and walking towards Castlemaine, will first go a

short distance down the compensation channel.'[14]
Bendigo Advertiser, Saturday 31 January 1874, p. 2.

'The open channel so frequently alluded to is constructed of masonry, and it leads the water for 180 odd feet [55 m] through a sluice-gate into the main channel which supplies Sandhurst, Castlemaine, Maldon, Fryerstown, and Taradale. ... At this point a compensation channel launches from the main to the old head of the Coliban River, and daily delivers into it half a million gallons of that water of which it has been deprived by the reservoir. By the side of the channel, and at the end of the embankment, a splendid waste weir pitched with bluestone has been provided, which satisfactorily accounts for any flood waters'.
The Sydney Morning Herald, Monday 1 February 1886, p. 6.

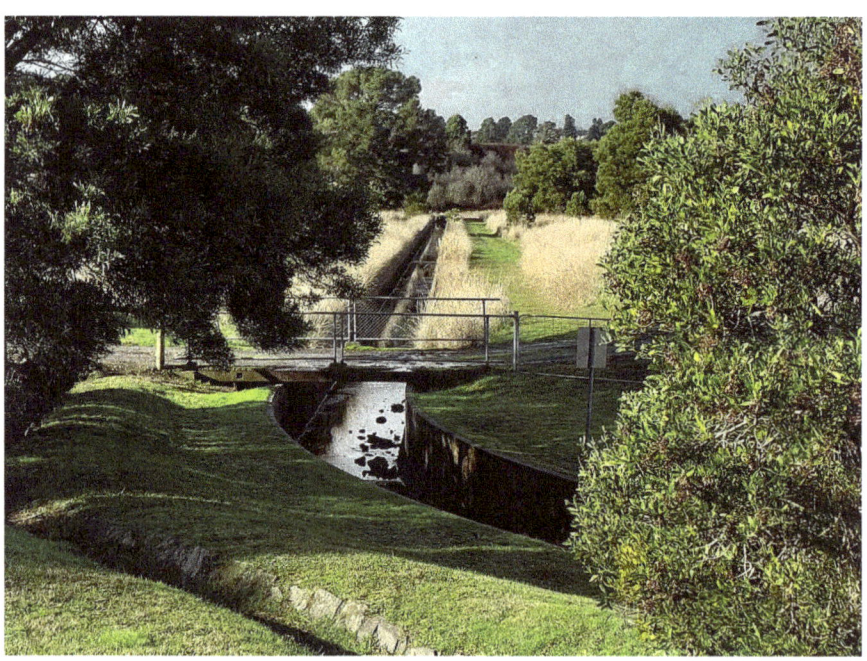

Start of the channel access track, Malmsbury.

---

14 The compensation channel is so called because water is allocated to the Coliban River to 'compensate' for flow that has been lost by being sent to Bendigo via the Main Channel.

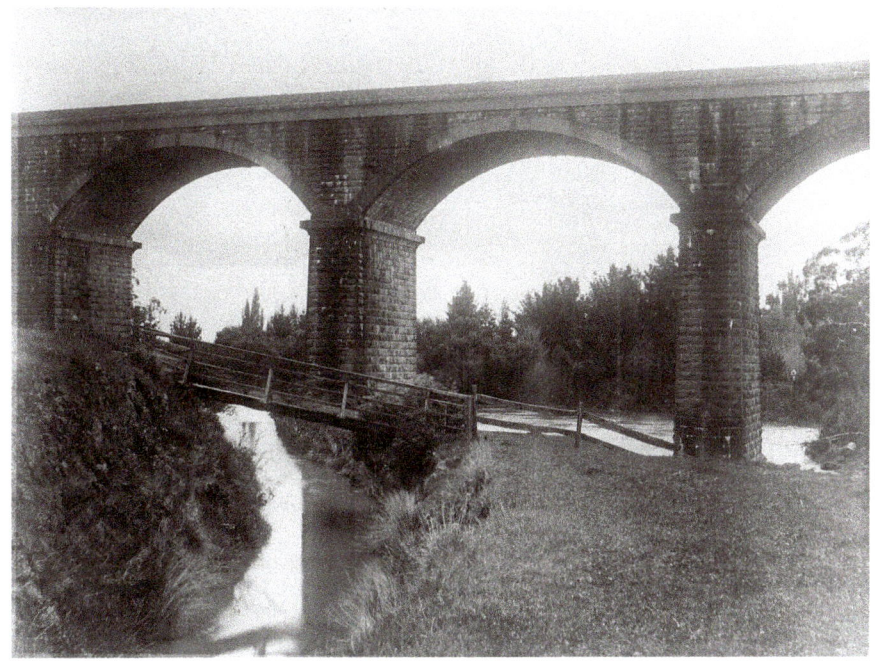

Viaduct, old channel, looking north.

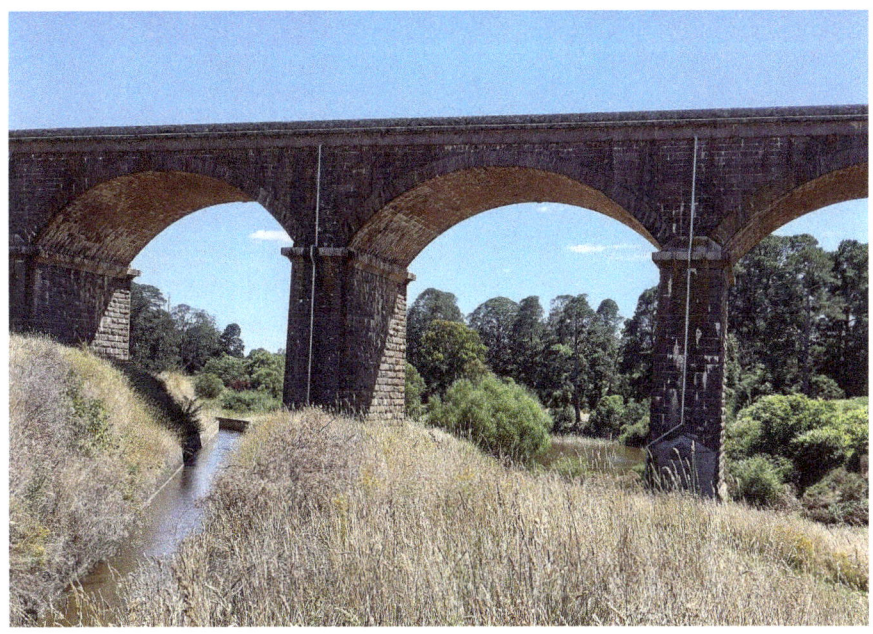

Present day view of the Malmsbury viaduct.

Heading north-east along the grassy track you will notice that the concrete race runs parallel to the original open channel (which runs to the west of the concrete race). Along many stretches of the Coliban channel you will see the old channel, built in the 1870s, diverge and head off in a different direction. There are some interesting historical artefacts within and beside the old superseded channel, but it certainly takes a lot of effort to view them. It's recommended that walkers on the outbound leg of this walk should stay on the main Coliban Channel access track.

About 500 metres into the walk you will pass under the Malmsbury Railway Viaduct. Built in 1859 to span the Coliban River, the viaduct is one of the largest 19th century bluestone structures in Victoria. It remains both an impressive sight and a significant engineering achievement consisting of five arched spans, 152 metres in length.[15]

After passing under the viaduct, the path follows the concrete race as it borders the Coliban River and the Malmsbury Botanic Gardens. It's worth making a detour to explore the gardens before

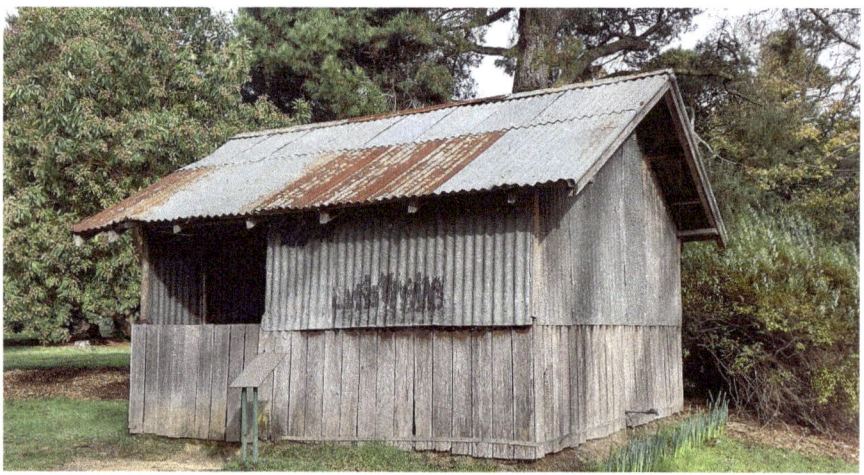

Fish hatchery, Malmsbury Botanic Gardens.

---

15 Quite possibly, the wooden bridge shown in the photo on the previous page also served as an overshoot designed to carry runoff across the channel. 'The floors of these shoots [sic] are laid transversely against the side-pieces of 9 x 1½ inch, with open joints immediately over the centre of the channel, to allow a certain amount of the drainage – where it comes off forest lands – to fall into the channel, and supplement the supply from the reservoir.' *Bendigo Advertiser*, 31 January 1874, p. 2.

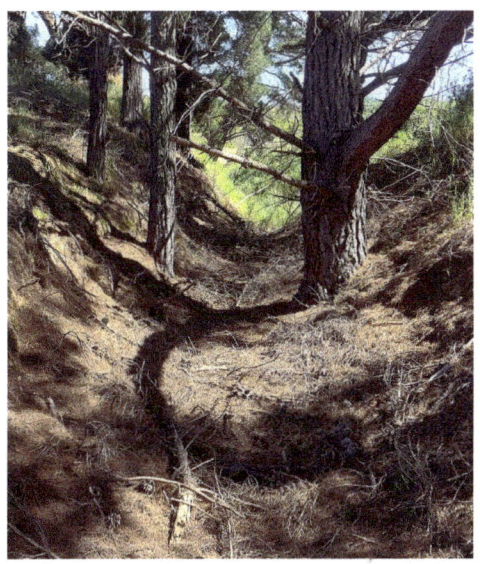

Original channel, Malmsbury.

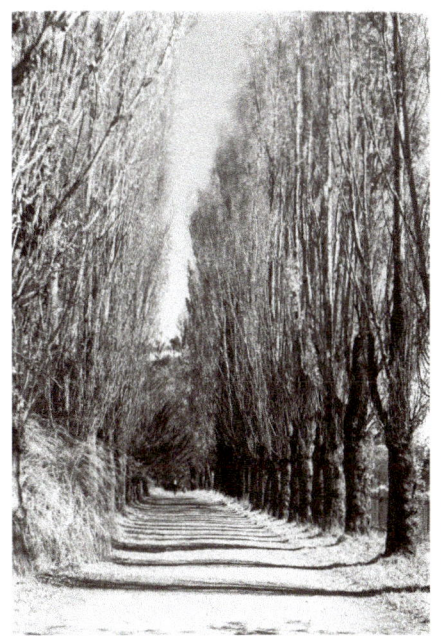

*The Gardens, Malmsbury, 1920s
(a vintage Rose Series postcard).*

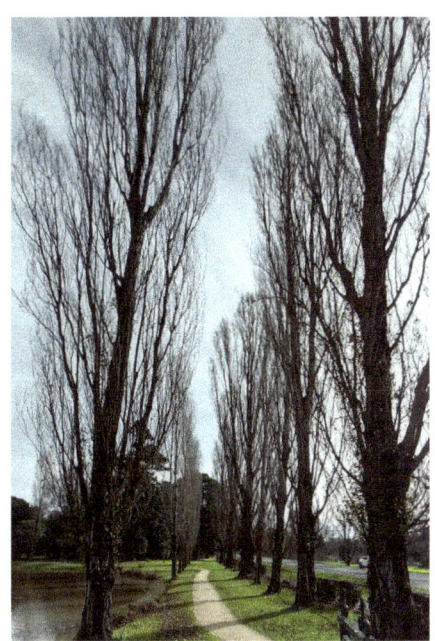

The same view today.

returning to the Coliban water race. Established in the 1850s, it is one of the earliest regional botanic gardens and has many old and notable trees. Within the gardens is a decommissioned fish hatchery which was used to rear trout between the 1890s and 1960s. Inside the hatchery is a stone well in which the fish were once kept.

After passing under the viaduct, to your left you will see the path of the old channel beyond some pine trees. Within a short distance beyond where the old channel meets the concrete race, you might be able to see the remains of an old brick weir (see photo below). The weir allowed water to be diverted to a side chute which led the water back to the Coliban River. It's all that remains of an early business venture designed to make use of the falling water to power a turbine which, it was hoped, would be used to saw through bluestone.

> 'The first attempt to utilise the Coliban water scheme for industrial purposes is being made at Malmsbury, where works for sawing bluestone into slabs for paving, etc., have

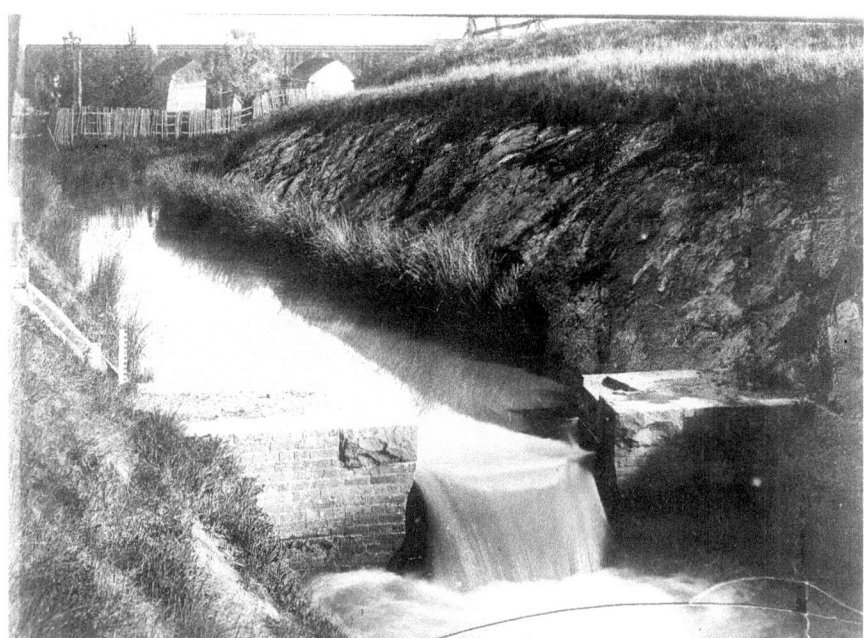

Old Malmsbury channel and brick weir. Note the entrance to a diversion channel leading to a turbine, above the weir on the left-hand side.

been erected by a company, the motive power for which is to be the water from the reservoir. ... The site is between the aqueduct and the river, a short distance below the railway viaduct. The works comprise four sets of frames of two saws each, but provision has been made for doubling the sawing power whenever it is requisite, as well as adding machinery for dressing and polishing granite and bluestone. A brick weir has been erected across the aqueduct, by means of which the water is diverted into a channel from which it falls into a well upon the turbine wheel by which the saws are worked, and is then conveyed by a discharge channel into the river, so that the company will be able to avail itself, if need be, of the full amount of compensation water allowed by the scheme for the river. The blocks of bluestone having been brought on drays from the quarries, are placed on carriages running on a tramway, and pushed directly under the frames which hold the saws. These saws are so counterpoised that, upon the machinery being put in motion, they exert on the stone just the necessary amount of pressure, cutting it at the average rate of one inch per hour.'
Bendigo Advertiser, 24 February 1874, p. 2.

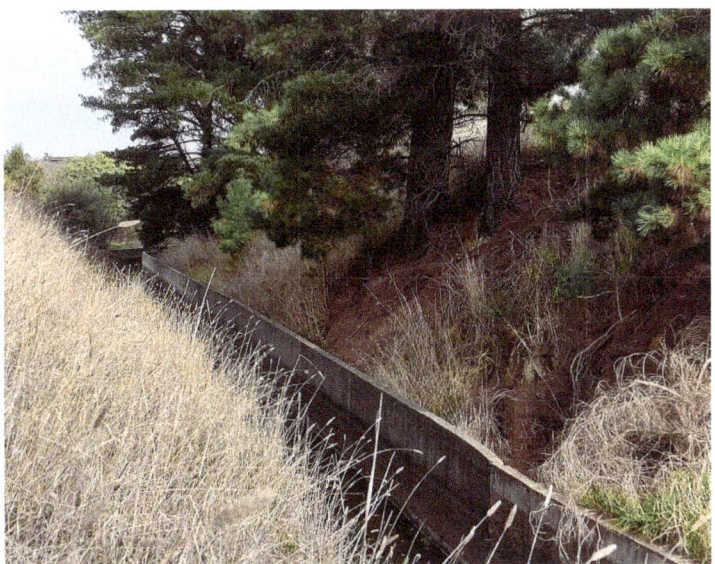

Present day view (remains of brick weir, bottom right-hand corner).

'Passing under the great railway bridge we come, a hundred yards further down, upon a mill that has been created for sawing bluestone in the same manner as it is sawn at Footscray with the difference that it is intended in this instance to utilize the compensation water as a motive power by means of a 23 h.p. turbine. The turbine is in its place, and everything prepared for the reception of the saws, but unfortunately a hitch has arisen about the supply of water. According to the statement of the directors of the company that is erecting the mill, Mr. Stone[16] promised to supply them with 1,112 cubic feet of water per minute, and finding that this quantity would drive a twenty-three horse power turbine, they put up their works accordingly. But it turns out that the compensation water allowed is, on an average, only about 140 cubic feet per minute, a quantity quite insufficient to drive the turbine. Mr. Stone's explanation, as I understand it, is that he was merely asked what quantity of water it would take to drive a twenty-three horse-power turbine, and having made a calculation replied that it would take 1,112 cubic feet per minute. There has evidently been a misunderstanding on one side, and blundering along in the dark on the other.'
Bendigo Advertiser, Saturday 31 January 1874, p. 2.

The brick culvert under the Calder Highway, known here as Mollison Street, is one of the many heritage listed structures along

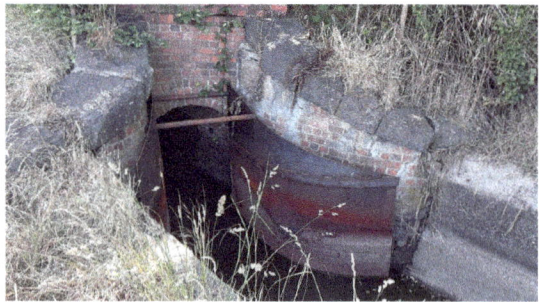

Culvert outlet under the Calder Highway, Malmsbury.

---

16 J.W. Stone was the local Victorian waterworks district engineer until 1876 when Mr. Henderson took charge of the completion of the Coliban Scheme. *The Age*, Wednesday 2 January 1878, p. 2.

the channel. It's now time to cross over the road and resume walking along the channel access track. Here to the left behind a row of trees is the now restored Blyth Brothers flour mill.[17]

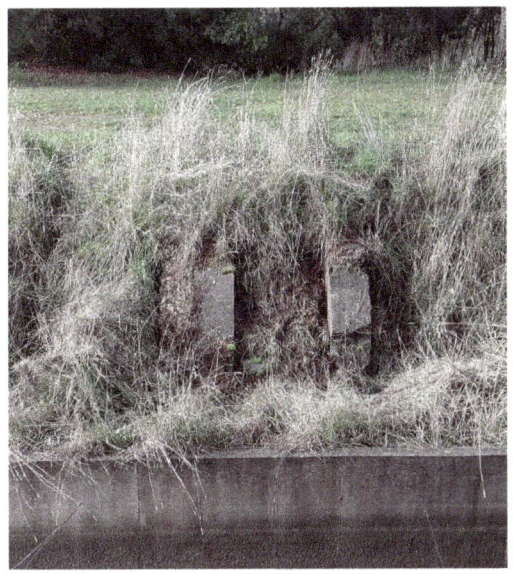

Remains of diversion channel to bluestone milling works.

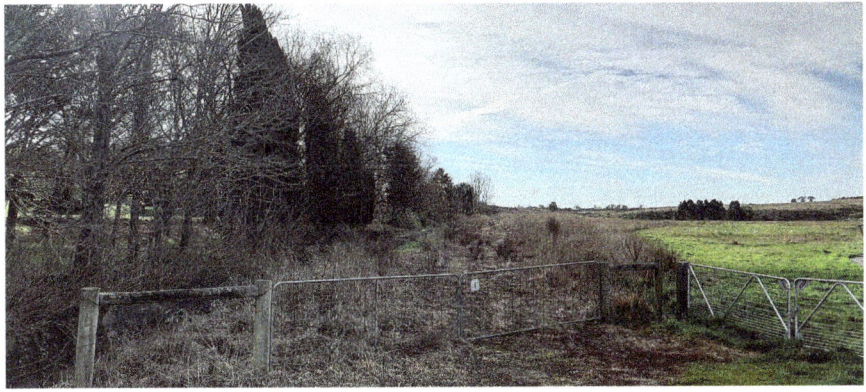

Channel access track north of Mollison Street, Malmsbury.

---

17 The Blyth Brothers flour mill was erected in 1861. It is now privately owned.

'Just as the channel leaves Malmsbury it passes, close to a deserted mill, the grounds of which are used as a camping place, and are littered with cattle droppings, old papers and the general refuse of a camp. The dust from this place and from the adjoining high road is no doubt blown into the channel by the wind, or partly washed in by the rain notwithstanding the overshoots which are here provided to carry the drainage water over the channel. From this point for some little distance northward the ground along the banks of the channel was let out for a small annual rental, not for grazing, but for cutting the grass ; there were, however, no signs of the grass having been cut, but there was ample evidence of grazing.'
Mt Alexander Mail, Saturday 29 May 1897, p. 2

'Before passing away from Malmsbury altogether, it may be interesting to know that the people of the little township, standing almost within the shadow of the great reservoir, can afford to laugh at the Coliban scheme, the streets being reticulated with beautiful water obtained from a spring on a neighboring hill'
Bendigo Advertiser, Saturday 31 January 1874, p. 2.

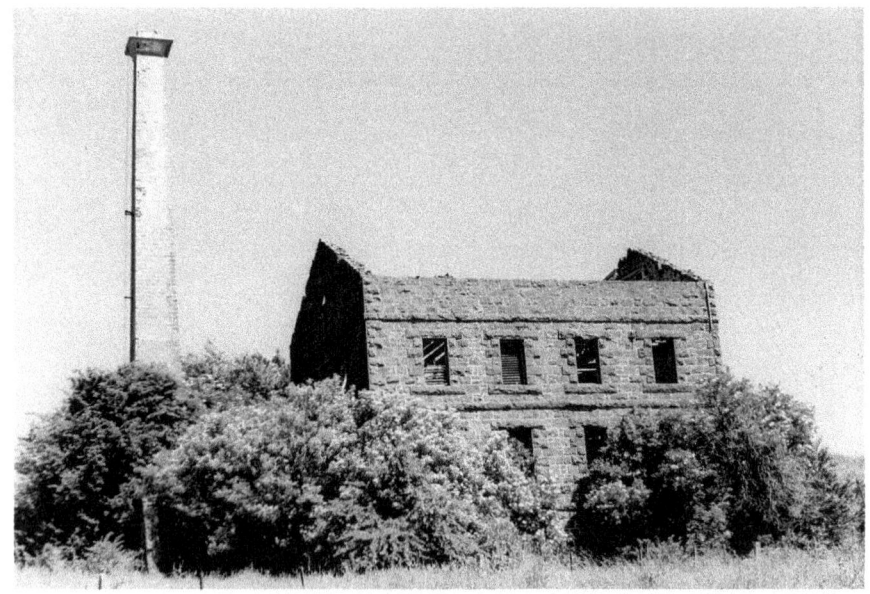

'Malmsbury Flour Mill' (photograph by John T. Collins, 1963-66)

'At the one-mile peg [1.6 km] a drain, which receives the rainfall and water from a slaughter-yard on the slope, above, empties itself into the aqueduct, and when the water in the channel is stirred up the stench, as might be expected, is abominable. All the shoots constructed in this vicinity are useless. They were intended to convey the drainage-water from the higher to the lower slopes across the aqueduct, but owing to defective design and construction they will not hold water, and no others are to be made.'
Leader, Saturday 31 January 1874, p. 20.

'To the left are the Malmsbury Flour Mills, the condensed water from which will be carried over the channel in a shute. Of these shutes, I may at once say, there will be altogether 48 along this section, the making of which will be let in small tenders of under £100 each.'
Bendigo Advertiser, Saturday 31 January 1874, p. 2.

'Further down the channel we found four heifers grazing within the reserve on the water's edge ; and at intervals along the whole length of the channel horse, cow, and dog dung were to be seen, and I was astonished to learn that the channel keepers were allowed to put each a horse and cow into the reserve to graze. But the most serious accumulation of animal refuse was

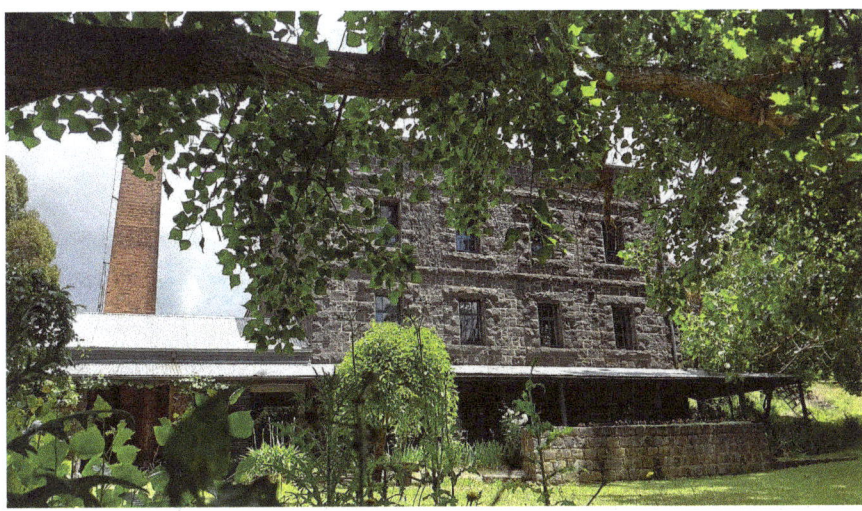

Present day view of Blyth Brothers mill.

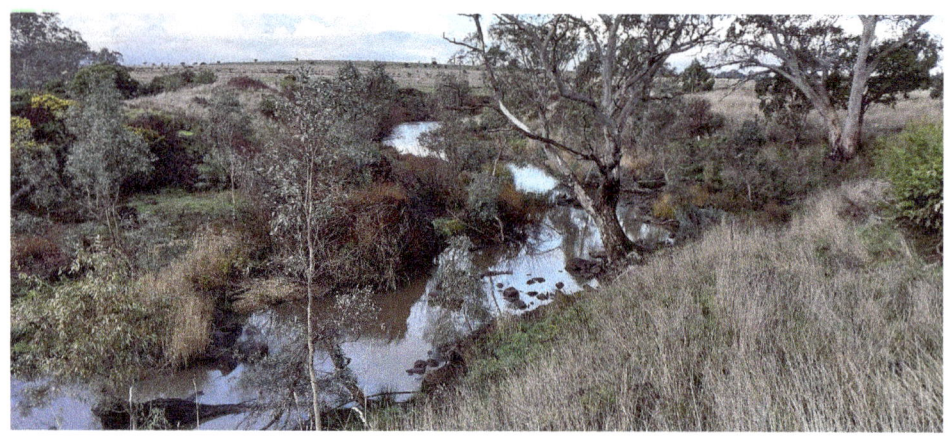
Coliban River, Malmsbury.

>the rabbit dung ; this was present along the greater length of the channel, and in some places the ground was thickly covered with it. Wire netting was fixed to the reserve fence in many places, but it was incomplete and too much out of repair to be of any use.'
>*Mount Alexander Mail, Saturday 29 May 1897, p. 2.*

Cattle are still encountered along some sections of the Coliban Water Channel access track. I've yet to encounter any that appear threatening, but it's wise to exercise caution when approaching them. Certainly it's important to close any gates that you have opened, and the gates have signs to remind you of that, but the majority of gates are locked and have to be climbed over.

>'The channel next passes for about 20 chains [402 m] through a heavy cutting in basalt, the greatest depth of which is 23 feet [7 m]. At 1 mile 20 chains [2 km], Brew's Gully is met with, the channel being carried over this by a pitched face crossing, lined with cement to a height of 2 feet 6 inches [762 mm], for a distance of about 3 chains [60.3 m]. At two miles [3.2 km, just beyond Forrest Road] there is a level crossing to be made, about 20 feet [6.1 m] of which will form a wide weir, for discharging the flood waters. This tender is also let. Thence to Boundy's Gully the channel is cut through basalt and scoriae.'
>*Bendigo Advertiser, Saturday 31 January 1874, p. 2.*

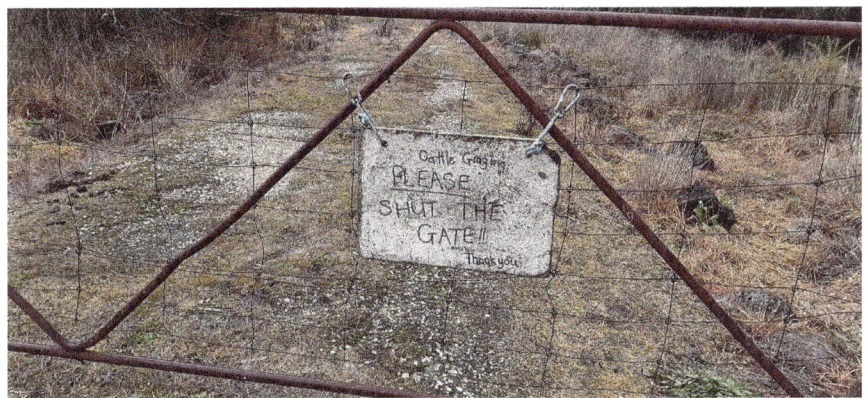
A gate along the access track.

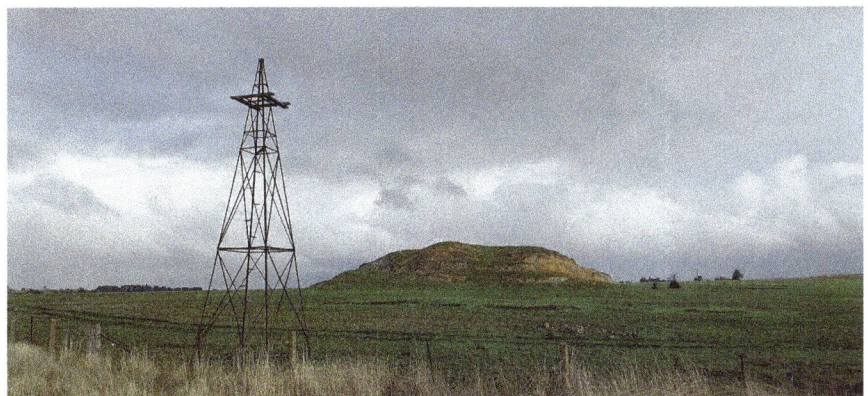
View southwards from the access track (mine spoil heap in background).

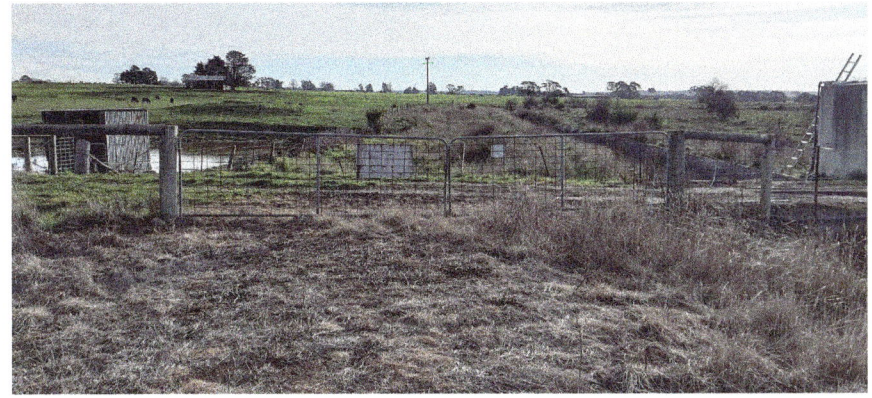
Forrest Road, furthest point for returning walkers.

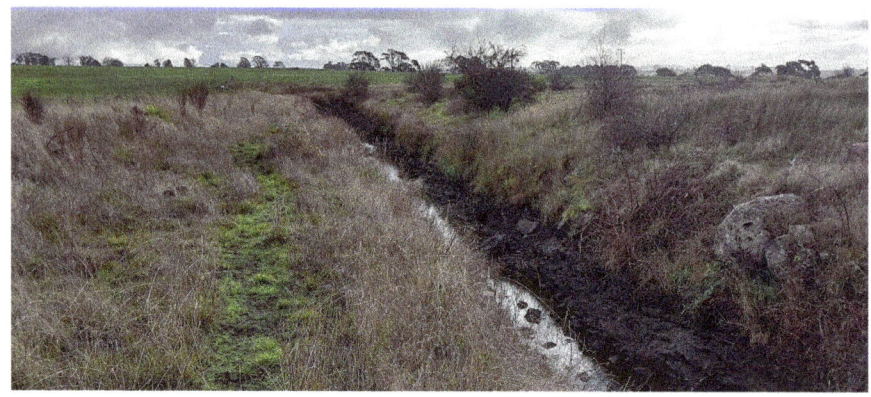
The channel reserve between Forrest Road and Boundy's Gully.

Forrest Road marks the end point for walkers who have parked at the Malmsbury Reservoir car park. You can choose to return the way you came or return via the alternative route already described (page 17). Those continuing on will need to climb over the gate here, making sure to avoid contact with the electric fence on the left-hand side of the gate. Once over the gate, walkers can either continue to pick their way along the reserve (B) which, until Forrest Road is met again and depending on the time of year, may well be overgrown and weedy, there being no marked track. The other option is to complete the walk to the Calder Highway via Forrest Road (A). Although Forrest Road is a minor road which carries little traffic, care should be exercised as there is no footpath bordering it.

Walkers who choose to walk on to the Calder Highway will cross over the channel again further up Forrest Road and pass by Boundy's Gully which is inaccessible as it is on private land.

> 'At Boundy's Gully the flume will be carried on a heavy rubble-work embankment which was built in Mr. Christopherson's time, and must have cost a large sum of money. Like all Mr. Christopherson's works in connection with this scheme it is substantial and splendidly made, but much too heavy and expensive for the purpose, which might have equally well been served by fluming carried on trestles. However, there it is, and, of course, Mr. Stone will take advantage of it to carry his flumes across the gully.'
> *Bendigo Advertiser, Saturday 31 January 1874, p. 2.*

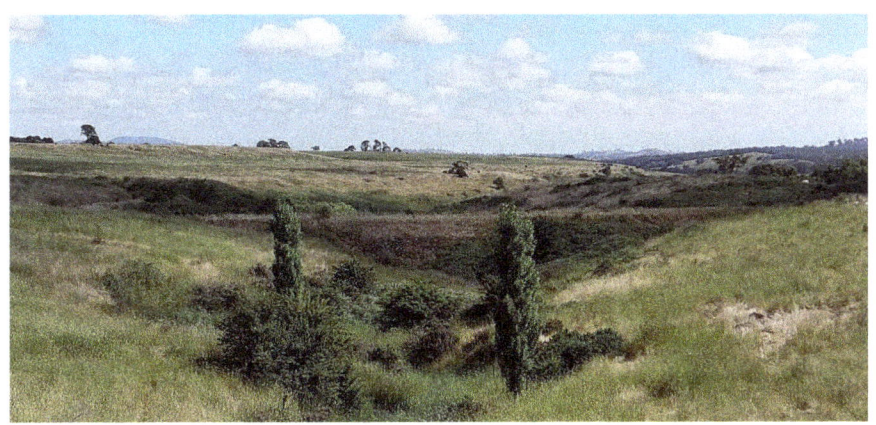

Boundy's Gully embankment from Forrest Road, looking north.

'That for some time past, there has been an extensive leakage of the main channel which takes the water to Castlemaine and Sandhurst, is well known around Malmsbury. The locality in which this occurs is about 2 miles from the township, to the right of the Mount Alexander-road. The race here crosses a deep but narrow ravine called Boundy's Gully by means of an earthen embankment. This leakage is not a new discovery. It has existed for a year or two in various forms without receiving much attention. At first the water was carried across by means of sheet iron fluming, but there are boys around Malmsbury, and it was one of their favourite diversions to throw heavy boulders into the flume, until by persistence and dexterity they thereby knocked several large holes into the bottom thereof. The department, finding that much of the water was running down the gully instead of reaching Castlemaine and Sandhurst, then erected an earthen embankment, which answered very well for a time.

A gang of men have been set to work to repair the Boundy's Gully leakage, and the water has been cut off since Saturday to

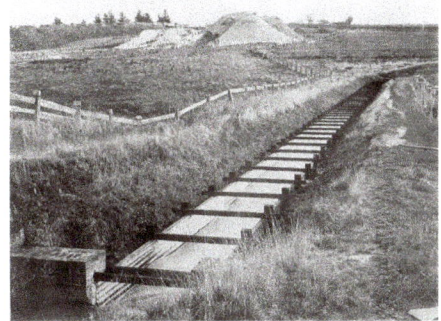

Flume at Boundy's Gully, 1893, looking west towards railway line (note the spoil heaps from mining operations).

enable this to be done. ... The design of the engineers who are carrying out the repairs is to enclose a corrugated iron trough soldered at the joints within an earthen flume which runs along the top of the embankment, and if this is done carefully it ought to be very effective. Since the water has been cut off there has been just sufficient liquid left stagnant in various depressed portions of the bed of the race to keep shoals of fish alive, and there they lay for a day or more at the disposal of anyone who comes to pick them up. Any number of fine English perch, some weighing 2 lb. and 3 lb., were thus obtainable. On Saturday night people were selling them about the streets of the borough at 6d. per bucket, and on Sunday crowds lined the sides of the race with heads bent and downcast eyes, ever and anon swooping upon stranded piscatorial prey'.
The Age, Tuesday 27 July 1886, p. 5.

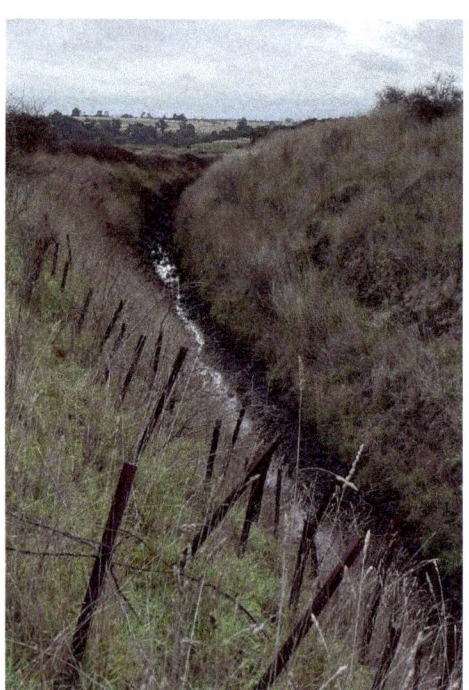

Channel between Boundy's Gully and No. 1 Tunnel.

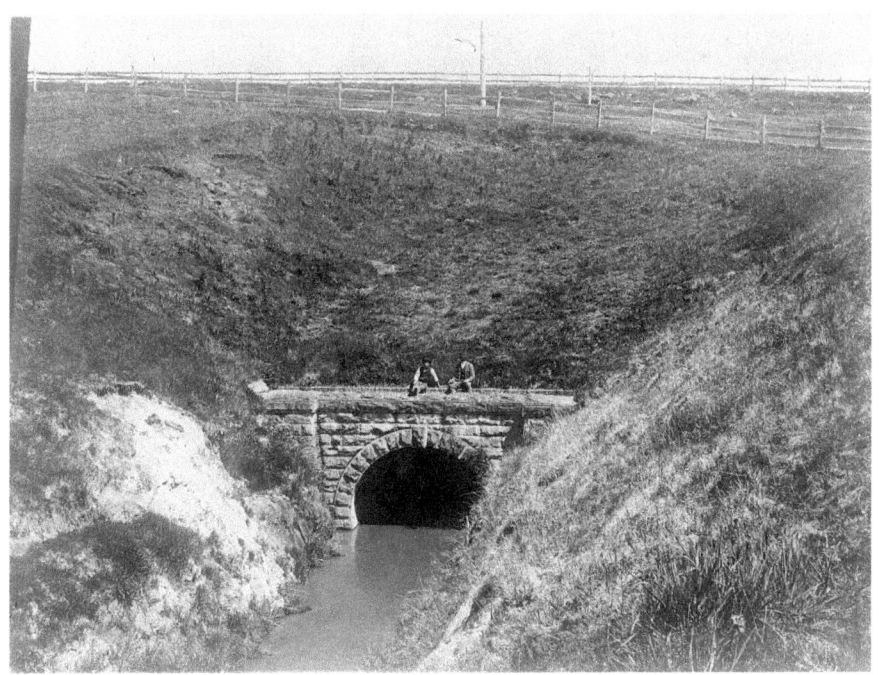

Entrance to No. 1 Tunnel.

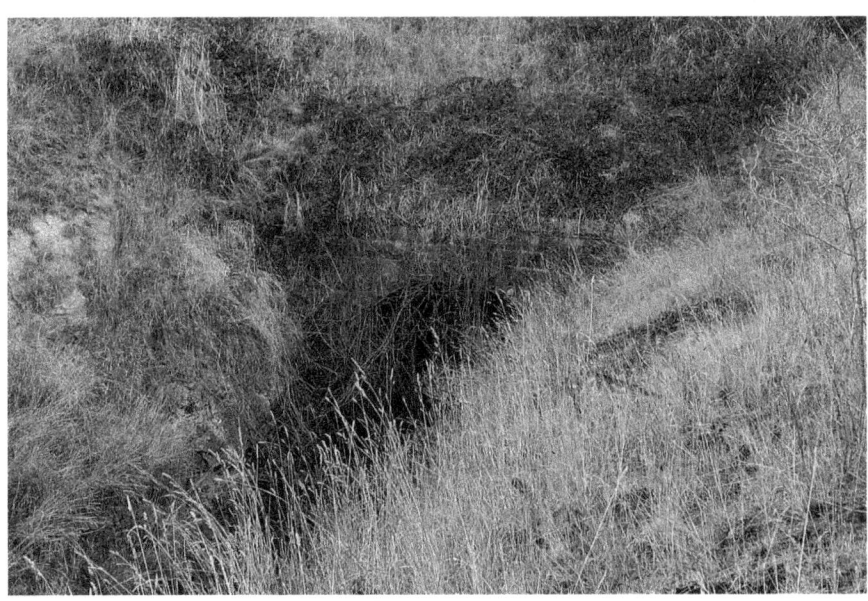

Present day view of above location.

'At 3 miles 10 chains [5 km] from Malmsbury — I forgot to mention that all distances are measured from the outlet channel— No. 1 tunnel- commences. It is ... 1825.5 feet [556 m] in length, driven through a formation of blue-stone boulders and clay, lined with brick cement. The sectional form adopted in No. 1, and all other tunnels along the main channel, is battered side walls, shallow curved inverts, and semicircular arch.'
Bendigo Advertiser, Saturday 31 January 1874, p. 2.

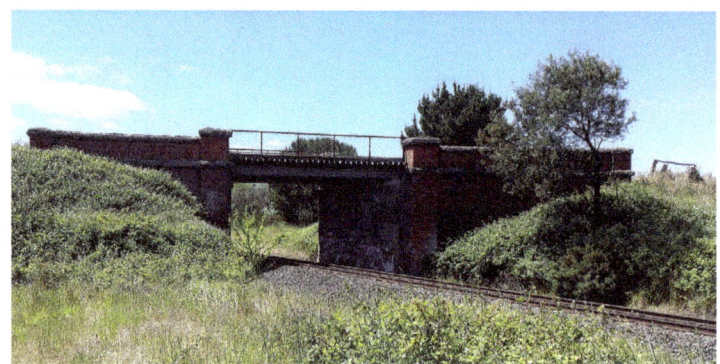

Forrest Road railway bridge.

'Well, as we can't conveniently pass through the tunnel, we must find our way over the hill, guided by the mounds of stuff sent up the shafts that were sunk along the course of the tunnel to facilitate its excavation. Descending the other side of the hill into the valley of the Back Creek, one can observe where, about half-way down, the bluestone, which has lasted all the way from Malmsbury, ends, and the schistose formation commences, the line of demarcation being very distinct.'
Bendigo Advertiser, Saturday 31 January 1874, p. 2.

The Back Creek Syphon

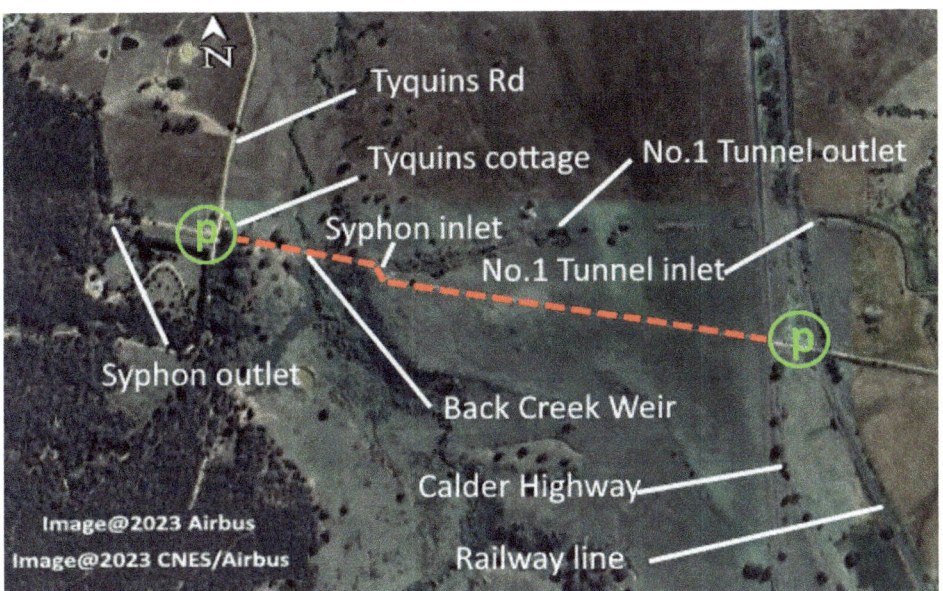

Back Creek syphon section (1.1 km).

The section of the channel between Forrest Road and the Back Creek syphon lies within freehold land and may only be walked with the permission of the landowner. Perhaps one day a similar arrangement will be made to that which allows walkers to traverse freehold land at Wirths and Brennans tunnels.

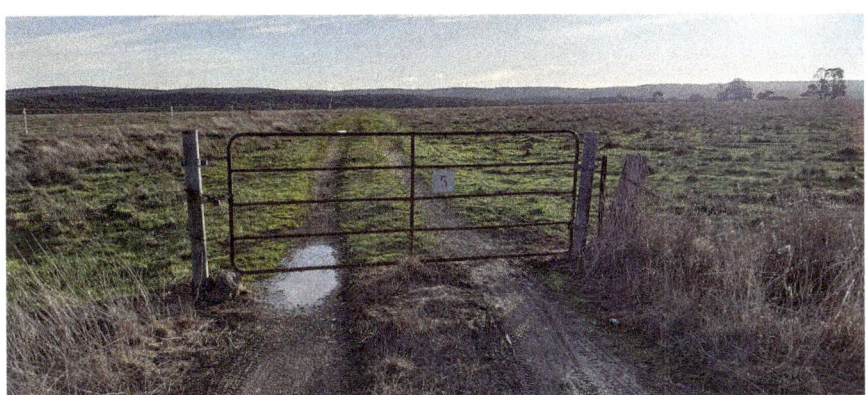

The Coliban Water access track to the Back Creek syphon inlet.

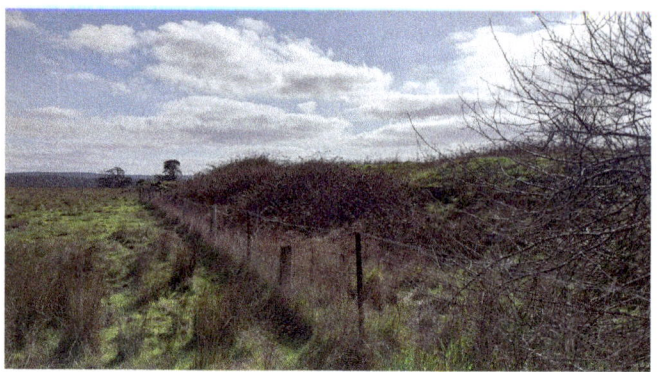

Line of spoil from tunnel excavations, Calder Highway.

Even if permission to tackle this linking section can be arranged, there are other problems to face. At intervals, cattle graze in the fields here. If so, it's probably inadvisable to disturb them.

Another difficulty is fording Back Creek if the creek is flowing fast. There's a concrete apron at the foot of the weir which might make a good bridge if dry. However, the riffle (stony shallows) just below the weir is probably a better option if there hasn't been recent heavy rain.

For those curious to know what the Main Channel looks like emerging from Tunnel No. 1, it's hardly worth the effort it costs to reach it. Either the original tunnel outlet has been demolished and replaced by this concrete pipe, or else it is lost beneath the mountainous blackberry thicket here. Further along, the Back Creek syphon inlet is reached, much altered in recent years.

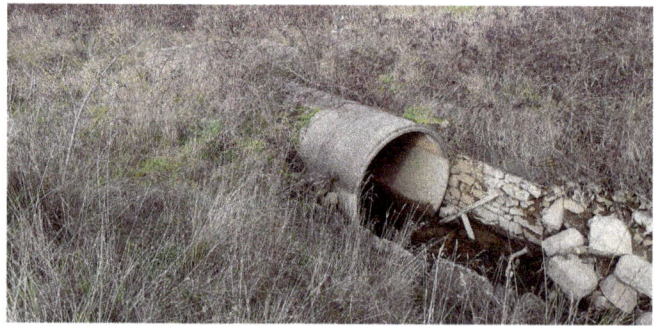

No. 1 Tunnel outlet (the old outlet is now removed or buried under blackberries).

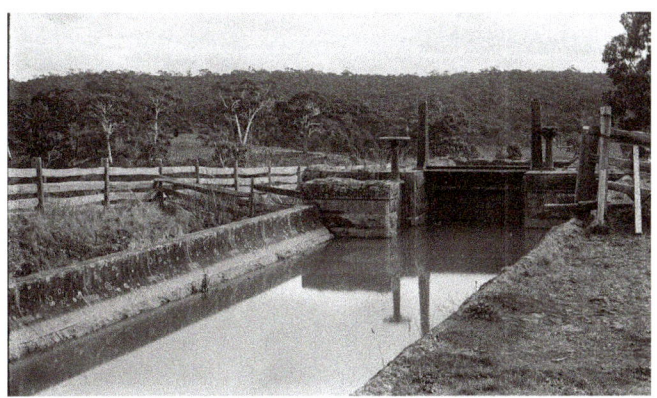

Back Creek syphon inlet (basalt-lined channel and regulator), 1940, SR&WSC.[18]

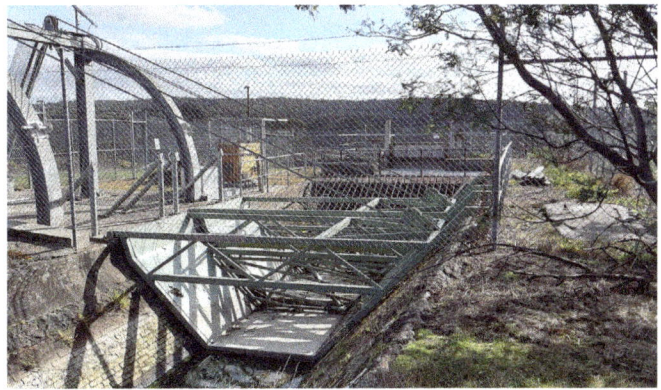

Present day view of Back Creek syphon entrance.

'Taradale will take its [town water] supply from Malmsbury. From a point about three miles and a half [5.6 km] along the main aqueduct large earthenware pipes are now being laid for a distance of a mile and a quarter to a service tank capable of storing 60,000 gal., from which Taradale will receive its domestic supply.'[19]
The Argus, Saturday 7 August 1875, p. 4.

---

18 The State Rivers and Water Supply Commission (SR&WSC) was created in 1905 as a result of bringing together all of the Victorian rural water trusts and irrigation schemes. The Commission survived for almost eighty years, being replaced by the Rural Water Commission in 1984.

19 It has been decommissioned.

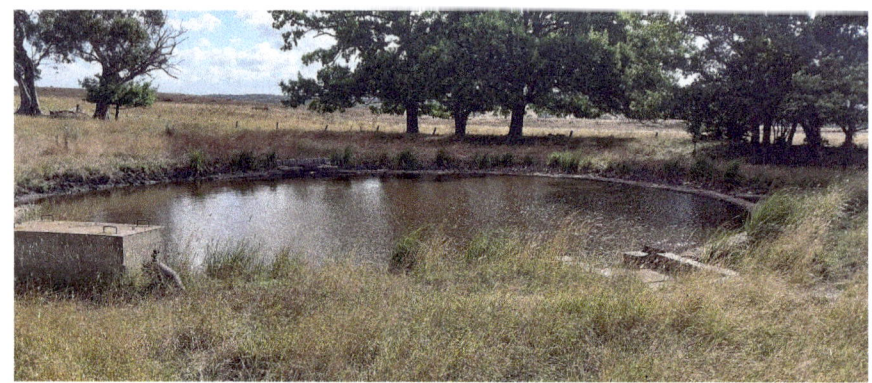
Remains of the Taradale Tank, near Conlans Road Taradale.

'First then, the supply is to be taken from the main channel, a few chains from the first tunnel which passes under the railway, and is nearly half a mile long-this was driven by Mr. Monie[20] – or at a point about 3.5 miles from the Malmsbury Reservoir. At this point a side sluice has been constructed on the lower bank of the aqueduct, which is raised or lowered by means of screw-gearing to any required opening, for the purpose of regulating the supply. The water is conveyed in earthenware pipes, about 15 inches [381 mm] in diameter, laid with an even or regular fall of, I am told, about 10 feet per mile, which, of course, necessitates a tortuous line, and passes across land purchased from Tucker and the London and Melbourne Mining Company. The length of this pipe-line is a little over a mile [1.6 km] to the service reservoir, and along it there is a well built every 200 yards [183 m] apart, to facilitate the clearing out of the pipes.

When necessary, these pipes cross gullies supported on timber beams, and the simple and inexpensive way in which this has been done was the subject of remark. The service reservoir is wholly in excavation, is circular, 70 feet [21.3 m] diameter, 6 feet [1.83 m] deep from grass; the bottom is formed with bluestone pitchers, laid dry; the sides of similar stone (looking rather rough, yet strong and serviceable), 5 or 6 feet high, and from the top of the masonry to grass there is an easy slope, springing from the back of the masonry wall, turfed to keep the water clean. There is also on the natural surface a kind of

---

20 The surname of this contractor is spelled three different ways in various newspaper reports.

table drain, about 10 feet [3 m] wide, apparently to keep out stormwater. There is also a well on one side for receiving the water from the earthenware pipes, and another on the opposite side for delivering the water to the town pipes, and valves and other contrivances.'
Bendigo Advertiser, Friday September 1 1876, p. 2.

The Failure of the First Back Creek Syphon

Along the course of the Coliban Main channel there are two gullies or valleys that were considered too difficult to bridge via wooden flumes. The first was the Back Creek valley, the second later became known as Whisky Gully on the eastern side of Mount Alexander. In both cases it was decided to carry the water across via a syphon.[21] As the photograph on page 44 shows,[22] an excavation was made to accommodate a pipe into which water enters from the open channel. Concrete walls, creating a weir, protect the syphon pipe at the lowest point of the valley. The syphon then rises up the other side of the Back Creek valley before emptying into the next section of open channel. As long as the exit point is lower than the entrance, water will flow across the valley.

However, the first Back Creek syphon was a complete and expensive failure. Journalists of the time had doubted the wisdom of using re-purposed Melbourne sewer pipes for this part of the project.

> 'The syphon is certainly a gigantic undertaking. In length, it is something over the third of a mile. Its lowest point – the creek level – is 100 ft below the inlet, and the fall from the inlet to the creek level is very abrupt, the declination being one in three, whilst on the other side the rise from the creek to the outlet is very gradual. The syphon pipe is composed of cast iron plates, each length consisting of four segments rivetted together by means of fishplates of wrought-iron. In fact, the syphon is constructed of the plates imported for the sewerage of Melbourne, the use of some of which for the outlet works at the Malmsbury Reservoir has been attended with such disastrous consequences ... It must be borne in mind that the castings were never intended for the use to which they have been put. They were never designed to bear inside pressure at all. It was never contemplated even that they would be made into a pipe of any

---

21 'Syphon' is an arcane spelling, nowadays it is usually spelled 'siphon'.
22 The photograph seems to show the 1874 syphon, built after the failure of the first.

kind. It was simply proposed that two of the segments should be joined together to form the arch of a brick lined sewer'.
Portland Guardian and Normanby General Advertiser, 1 Dec 1870, p. 5.

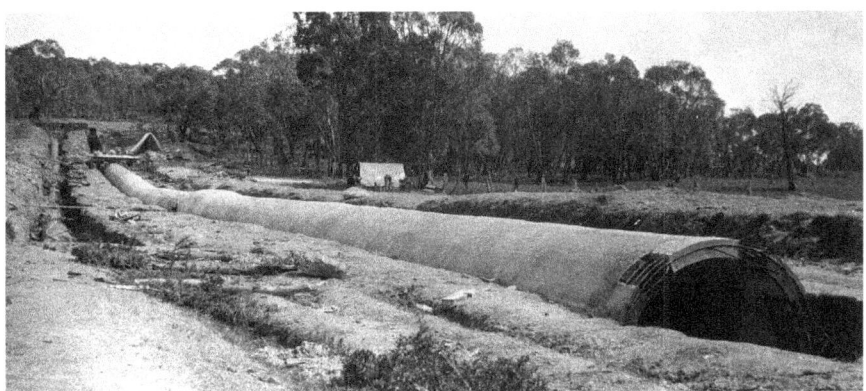

Back Creek syphon, 1930 (replacing an older decommissioned syphon on left).

Unfortunately these pipes proved to be as unsatisfactory for this purpose as their use as an outlet pipe at Malmsbury Reservoir.

> 'When the water was allowed to fill into the inverted syphon constructed in this manner the pressure became much too great for its power of resistance, and plate after plate fractured. As fast as one plate was replaced others gave way immediately the water was turned on into the syphon, and at last the attempt to carry water across the Back Creek by means of this peculiar iron piping had to be abandoned'.
>
> 'The fact was the pipes in question were ordered and designed for Melbourne sewage purposes, but as they had not been employed for that work it was thought they might be used in making the Back Creek syphon, but a more egregious blunder, as experience proved, was never committed. For these and other reasons several officers were suspended, and the works were for some time left in abeyance...'
> *The Age, 2 January 1878, p. 2.*

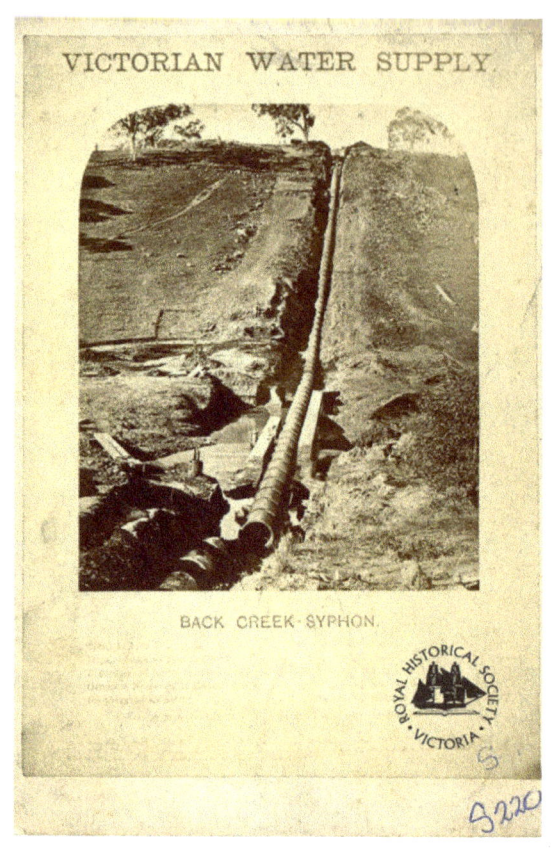

Second Back Creek syphon 1874.

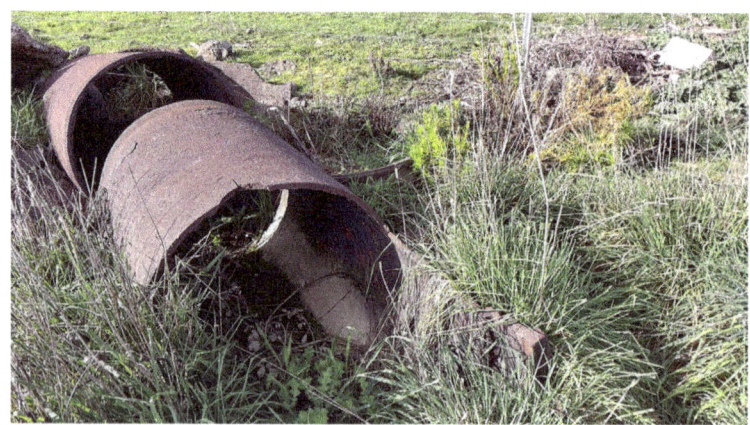

Remnants of an earlier syphon?

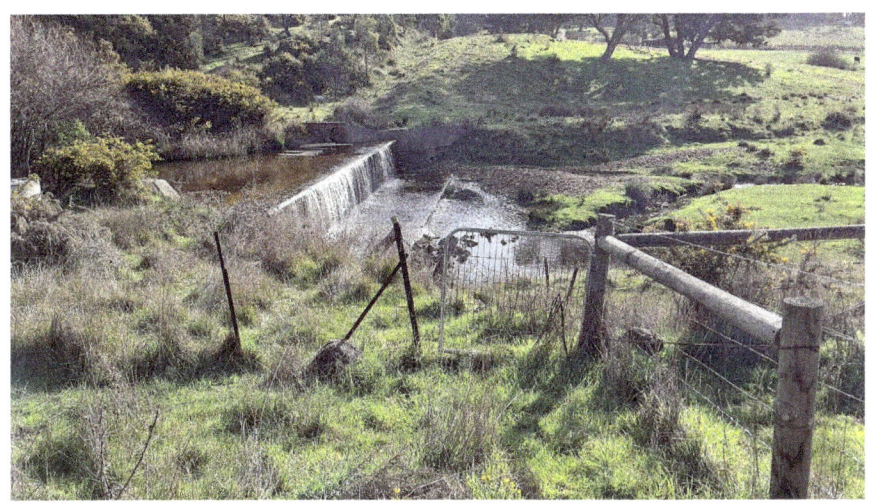

Approaching the Back Creek weir.

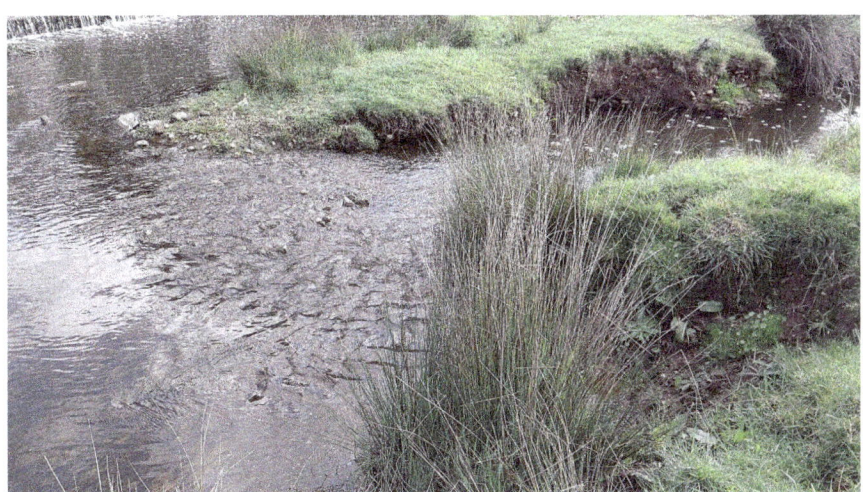

Crossing point on Back Creek.

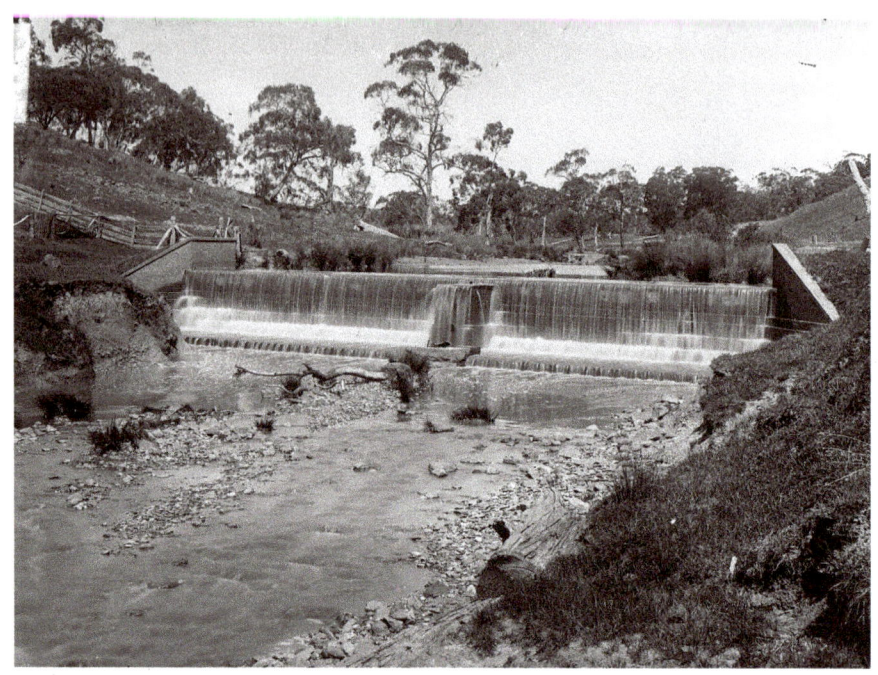

Back Creek syphon weir, 1938.

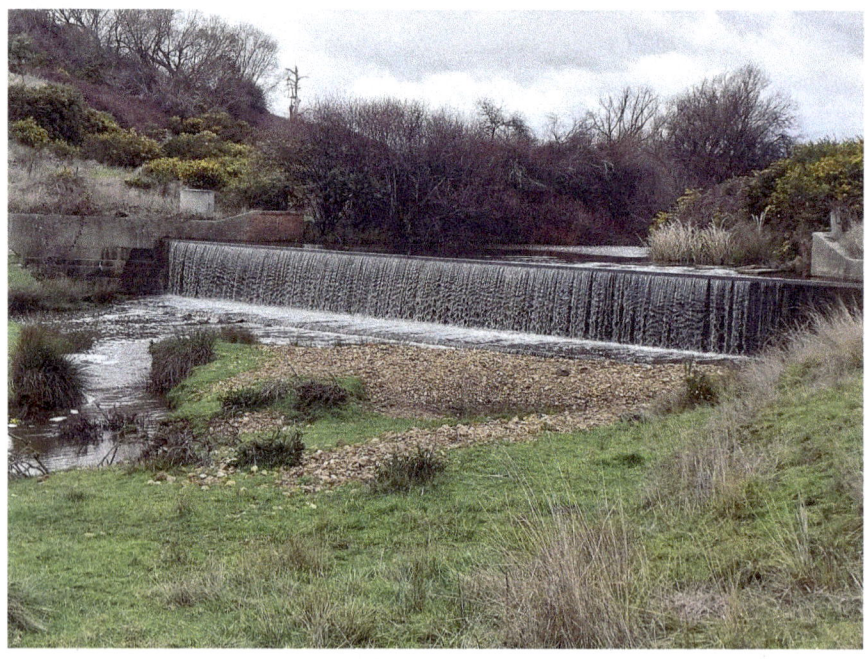

Present day view, Back Creek weir.

Back Creek Syphon Outlet to Taradale Road

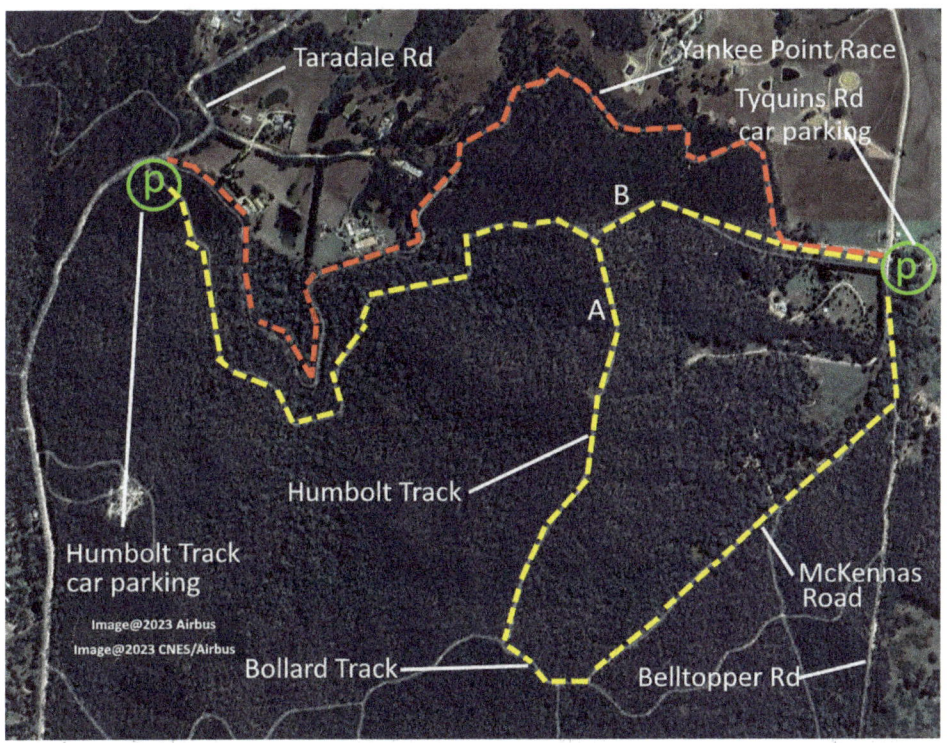

This walk is quite easy if walkers keep to the formed access track and roads. Those who are using a car shuttle can park off Tyquins Road near the Back Creek syphon easement or in the parking area near the intersection of Taradale Road and Humbolt Track. This seven kilometre return walk begins near Tyquins Cottage.

A number of these sections (on maps, the red dashed outward bound paths) can be combined if a car shuttle can be arranged to create a more challenging day walk.

Along the channel at regular intervals, channel keepers were appointed to maintain the channel and perhaps monitor and charge for water usage where sluices were constructed. They later became known as water bailiffs. Many of the original keepers' houses have been demolished or relocated. However, the location

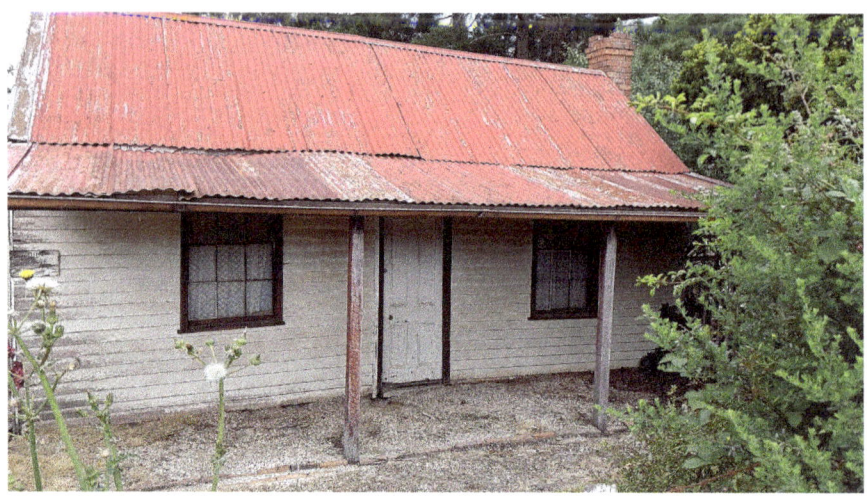
Tyquins Cottage, Back Creek syphon.

of Tyquins cottage at the start of this section and adjacent to the Back Creek syphon suggests it might have once had that function. Malcolm Phillips, a descendent of the original landowner, told me the house was built in 1874, which corresponds very closely to the year of construction of the other early channel keepers' houses.

Walk up the hill along the syphon easement. At the top, the outlet of the syphon will be encountered. This is heritage listed. It hasn't been much altered in 150 years. The channel access track can now be followed to Taradale Road.

About 890 metres downstream from the outlet, keep an eye out for the Yankee Point race. This was cut in March 1875 by R. Jamison and party to provide water for sluicing.[23]

> 'About four miles and a half [7.2 km] from Malmsbury, on the northern side of the Back Creek syphon, a race has been cut to Yankee Point, Taradale, to supply some large claims there. The department is selling 18,000 gal. an hour to the miners there'.
> *The Argus, Saturday 7 August 1875, p. 4.*

> 'For a considerable time there has been a suspicion that the puddling-machine of Miller Brothers at Yankee Point, Taradale, was visited in the night-time and robbed. A watch has been set

---

23 *Mount Alexander Mail*, 6 March 1875, p. 2.

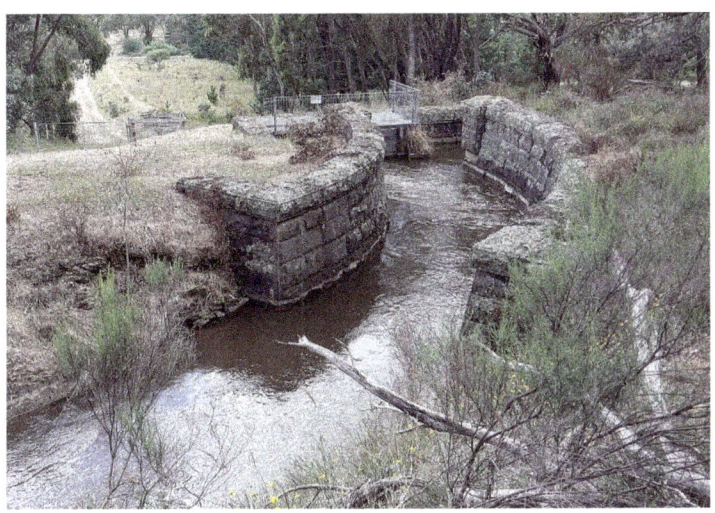

Back Creek syphon outlet.

for more than a week. Constable Brunker taking his turn with the proprietors of the claim, four in number, who watched two and two. At 2 o'clock on Monday morning the Miller Brothers, who were on watch, saw an old miner named Enoch Simms approach with a number of tools and a lantern.[24] Simms pulled the stoppers out, letting the water that was in the bottom of

> **TARADALE.**
> (FROM OUR OWN CORRESPONDENT.)
> May 15th, 1856.
> I took a stroll yesterday morning through the once busy regions of Yankee Point and Liberty Flat. What a considerable contrast it presented to its former stir and bustle. The ground, which a month ago was literally covered with an active population, and where the merry ring of pick and shovel was daily heard, is now solitary and almost deserted. Here and there it is true, a care-worn digger may be seen, screwing his courage to the sticking place, patiently suffering the ills that are by turning out four buckets of water to one of dirt, rather than rush into a seventy feet duffer and endure greater.

---

24 Liberty Flat and Yankee Point were sites of feverish fossicking in the 1850s but, like many other areas in central Victoria, were quickly worked out and deserted. Nevertheless, mining operations continued on and off over the years. In this case, water from the Coliban Channel reactivated the search for gold.

the machine off. He then cleaned up the sluice boxes, putting the cleanings in a can for removal, replacing sand and stones in the boxes to destroy his traces. He then got into the machine to clean that up, and was arrested by the two Millers in the very act. He was bound and handed over to Constable Brunker, who placed him in the lock-up. Simms was brought before Mr. Dunbar, J P., and remanded to the Castlemaine Gaol until 7th inst'.
Argus, Wednesday 4 September 1895, p. 6.

Not far from Taradale Road there's an 'orphaned' vestige of the channel. These old bypassed sections are worth visiting as they show how the original channel once looked.

At Taradale Road turn left and return to Tyquins Cottage via Humbolt Track, Bollard Track and McKenna's Track (yellow line A). There is an option of taking a shortcut (yellow line B) but good navigation skills (aided by a GPS app) are needed, first to find the place to divert from Humbolt Track (at the point where the Track turns sharply south), and then to navigate back to

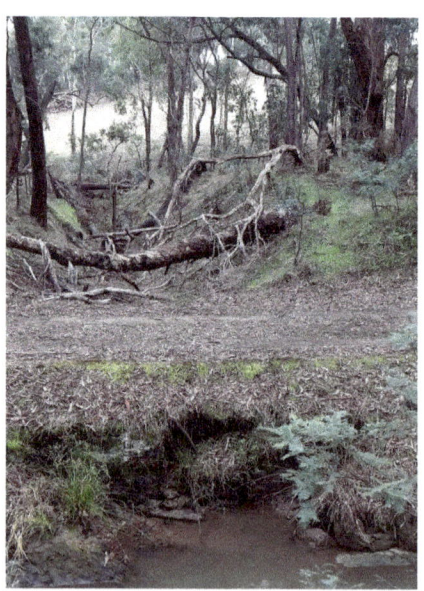 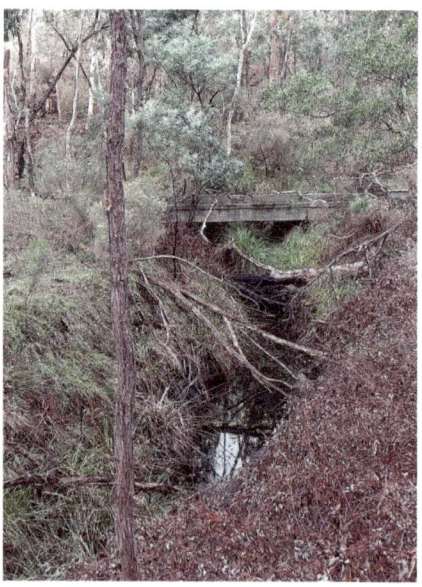

Start of Yankee Point race, Taradale, culvert in foreground. Right: Old Coliban Channel near Taradale Road.

Tyquins Road. There is a steep gully in this section, and once you climb out of this gully, and if you've been keeping an easterly line, you should encounter a fence. Stay to the left of it and it will lead you back to the Back Creek syphon outlet.

It should be pointed out that walkers will likely encounter snakes all along the channel, especially during spring and summer. It pays to keep one eye on the path in front of you. Red-bellied black snakes and tiger snakes are those most commonly seen, but all move quickly away if given half a chance.

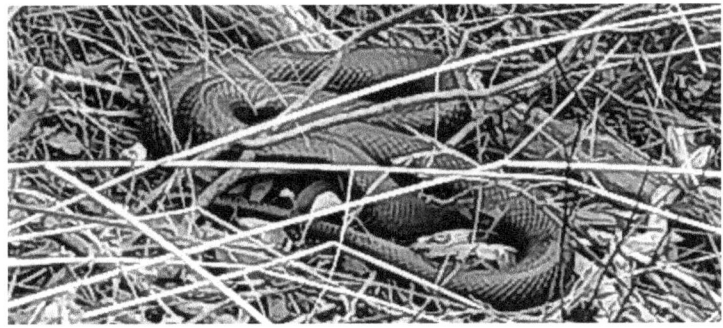

Red-bellied black snakes.

Taradale Road to Fryerstown Road

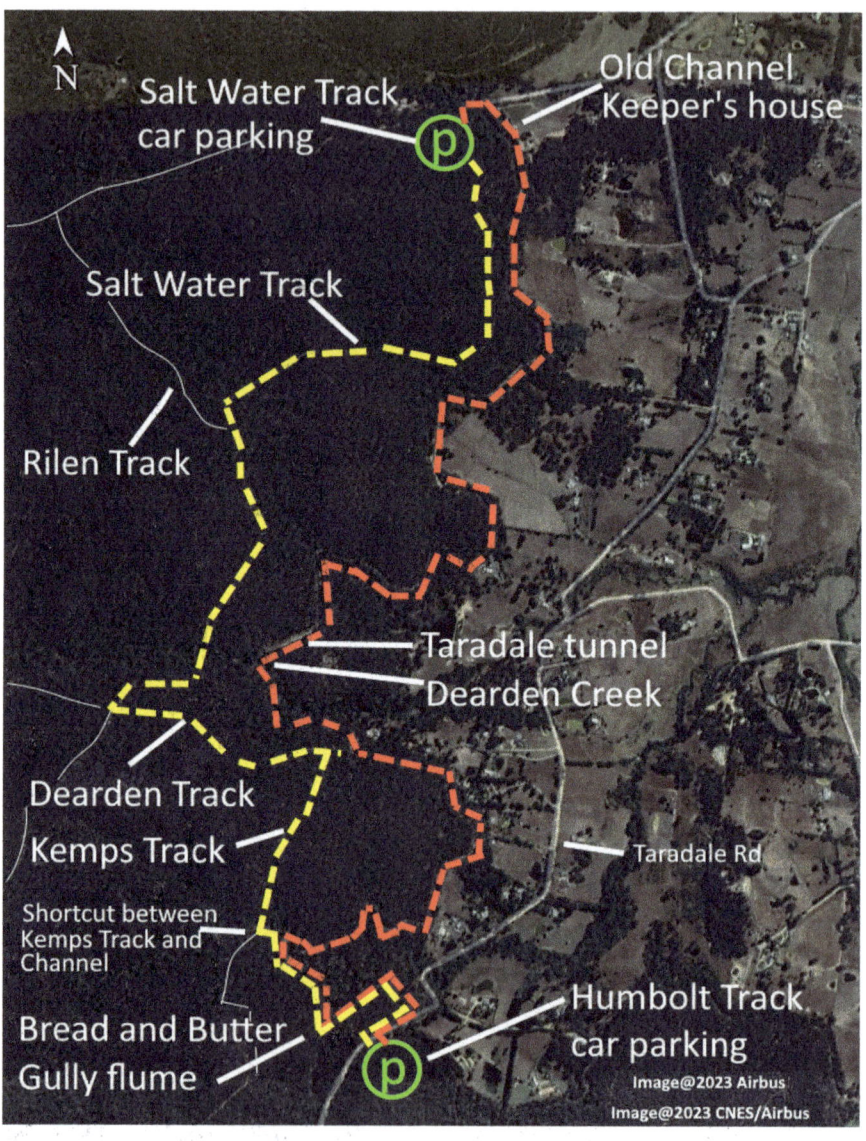

As in the previous section, a return walk of about 11 km can be made by using roads that run roughly parallel to the channel, in this case, Salt Water Track and Kemps Track. Those having the option of a car shuttle can park just off Humbolt Track near its intersection with Taradale Road, with the second car parking off Salt Water Track near its intersection with Fryerstown Road.

So begin by turning right at Taradale Road and left onto the Coliban Channel access track. Soon you will reach an interesting feature which is off the main track, about 400 metres from the starting point. Instead of descending the track at the tree fern gully here, continue to follow the channel to the left. Within a hundred metres you'll arrive at Bread and Butter Gully which is the site of a historic flume which has been altered over the years (not least, sadly, by graffitists) but the original flume abutments are still visible.

Bread and Butter Gully must once have been beautiful, with resplendent tree ferns, some of which survive today. There's a handrail for those courageous enough to walk across the concrete flume. However it's definitely safer to return the way you came and pick up the access track again. For those who have crossed the flume, you'll rejoin the access track in about 70 metres.

> 'Turning our backs upon the Back Creek, we resume our journey along the bank of the channel. Bread and Butter Gully, six miles, will be crossed by an iron and trussed timber flume on brick piers. The piers are built, and the contract let for the fluming."
> *Bendigo Advertiser, Saturday 31 January 1874, p. 2.*

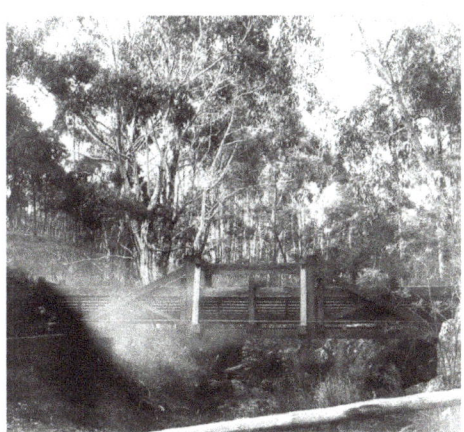 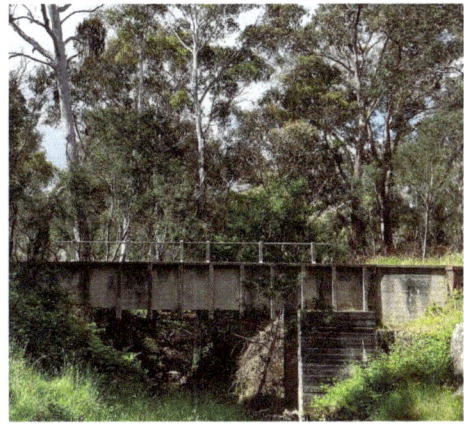

Original timber flume at Bread and Butter Gully. Right: Present day view.

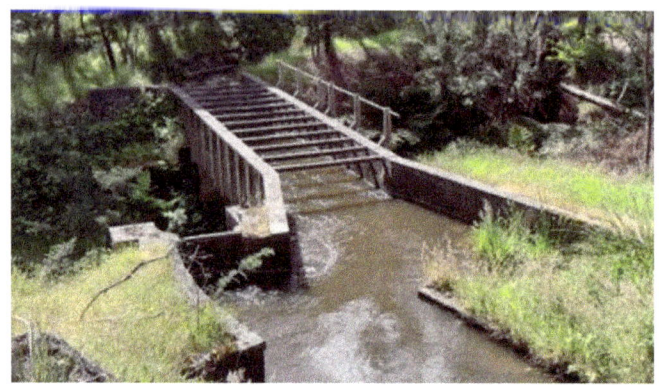

Bread and Butter Gully flume (note old abutments on the left).

About 400 metres further on you'll encounter a large culvert and weir at Kangaroo Creek.[25] There are a number of these structures along this section of the channel. They appear to be very efficient engineering solutions to spanning creek beds. The water is channelled through a pipe while side stream floodwaters are directed over the top to continue their journey downstream.

Originally, this culvert and weir was a corrugated iron flume. The brick abutments can be seen in the photo (page 55) on the right-hand side.

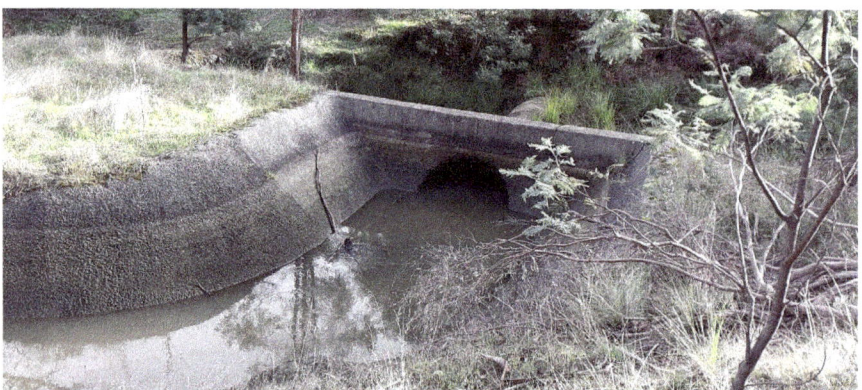

Culvert and weir, Kangaroo Creek, site of a shortcut to Kemps Track.

---

25 To confuse matters, there are two Kangaroo Creeks along the Main Channel in Taradale. In this case it's the creek just north of Taradale Road. The other Kangaroo Creek crosses the Channel near Salt Water Track in the north.

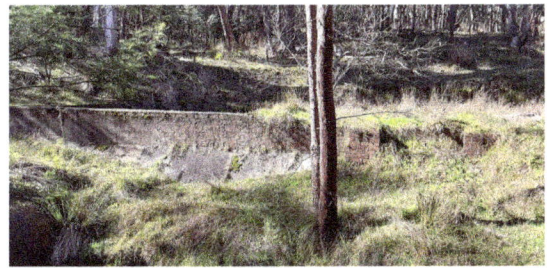

Old corrugated iron flume abutments (RHS).

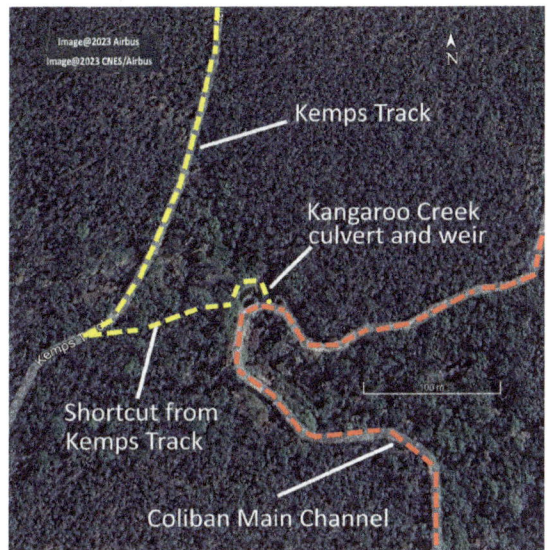

Close up of a shortcut to Kemps Track (yellow path).

If you intend to do the return walk, it might be easier to do so in a clockwise direction and return via the channel, as it's tricky to find the above shortcut if approaching from Kemps Track. Head over the weir and then pick up a foot trail which should be followed until you reach Kemps Track (see photos above). Turn right, cross the Kangaroo Creek Gully and follow Kemps Track 620 metres to Dearden Track. Turn left, continue on for 700 metres and then turn right at Salt Water Track. Follow this until you reach Fryerstown Road.

For those not leaving the channel, continue to walk along the access track. After crossing Dearden Track, another culvert and weir is encountered in 470 metres at Dearden Creek.

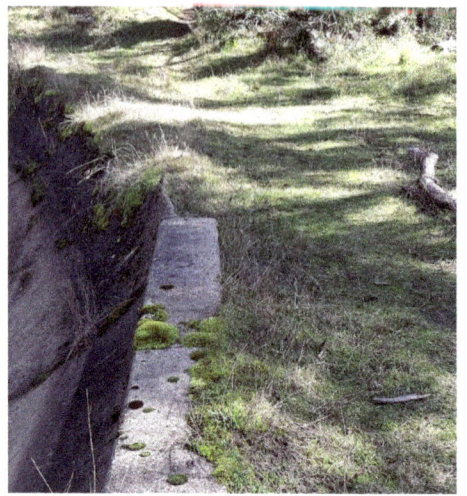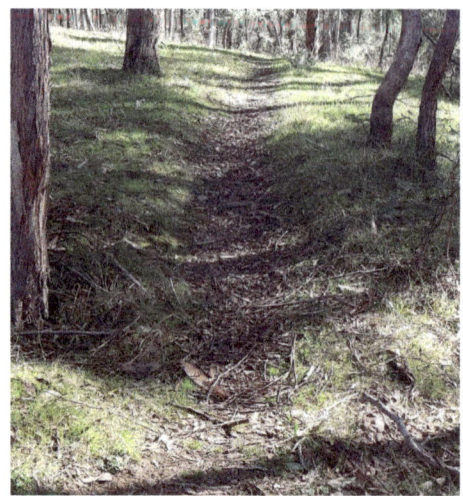

Walking Path from the channel to Kemps Track.

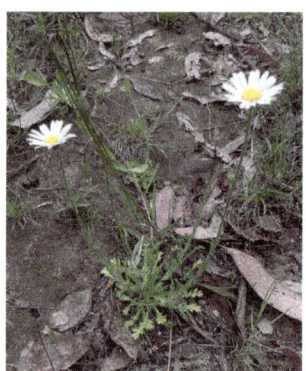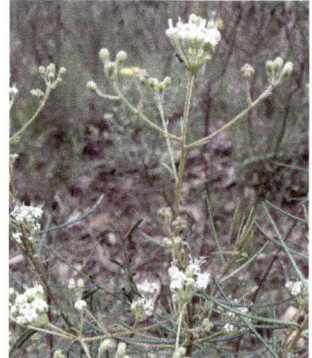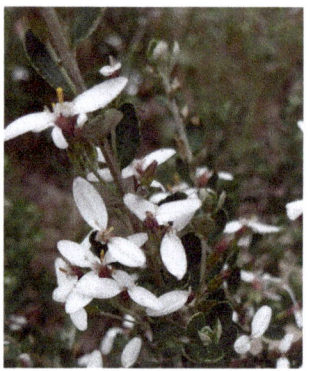

Tall daisy.　　　　　*Rough star-hair.*　　　　*Silky daisy-bush.*

Along this section of Coliban Channel a number of less commonly seen wildflowers grow. If walking in the springtime keep an eye out for these plants which have restricted ranges within this region.

With the near collapse of the Malmsbury Reservoir embankment and the necessary redesign and reconstruction of the Back Creek syphon, work came to a halt on the Coliban Water Scheme. When work finally resumed in 1874 a sad sight met the returning workers along the channel, in particular just north of Dearden Track where a cutting had collapsed and couldn't be easily re-excavated.

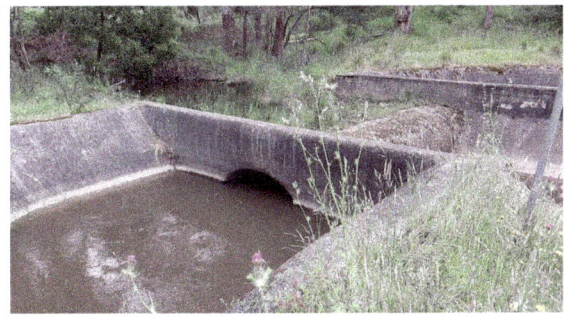
Culvert and weir at Dearden Creek.

> 'At 73/4 miles [12.5 km], in a very deep cutting, there has been an enormous slip from the eastern bank of immense granite blocks, which might possibly have been averted had the watertable been sooner cut. It would be very difficult to raise the blocks out of the cutting, and, therefore, a contract to tunnel through the slip, a distance of 132 feet [40.2 m], has been let'.
> *Bendigo Advertiser, Saturday 31 January 1874, p. 2.*

Although this tunnel was constructed when work resumed on the channel, it wasn't given a number, as was the case with all the other tunnels along the channel route. Perhaps this was because numbers had been allocated in the early design stage of the scheme.

> 'The main channel was completed as far as the 18th mile in September, 1874. Up to that point it has cost £126,000. There is nothing in the appearance of the works to justify the expenditure of such an enormous sum, so far as an unprofessional eye can judge. Of course £23,000 of the sum total was absolutely thrown away over the ridiculous exhibition of engineering folly at the Back Creek, and it is patent to any observer that the channel is unnecessarily tortuous, and that some of the principal works upon it, notably the tunnel[s] are far from being specimens of economical construction. Had more care been originally taken in laying out the channel, … less steep and heavy excavations would have been required in many places, and it is believed that a saving of something like four miles in a length of 20 miles of channel would have been made'.
> *The Argus, Saturday 7 August 1875, p. 4*

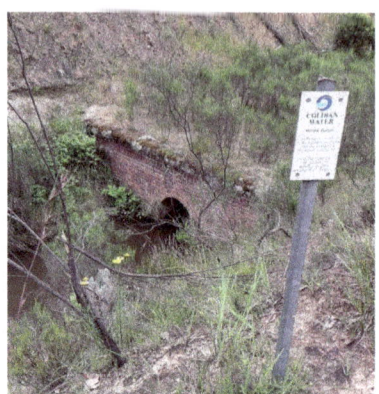

Taradale tunnel inlet, present day view.

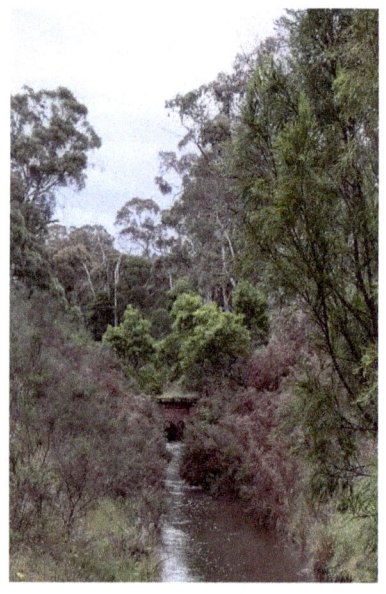

Taradale tunnel exit.

'Culverts and weirs are used where the gullies or creeks, crossed by the channel, have an insufficient fall on the lower side of the line to allow of the drainage being taken under the floor of the channel. The culvert which takes the channel water is of the same form as those already explained, with segmental formed wing walls at both sides, built in concrete, and extended into the side slopes for a distance of 20 feet, and carried to a height of 3 feet above the crown of the culvert.

The stormwaters coming down the creeks will be impounded by these means to a sufficient height to allow of a fall into a pitched basin on the lower side of the culvert, whence they will escape into the old creeks. There are three of these combined culverts and weirs, all situated on the line of extensive drainage areas, and capable of discharging from 300 to 500 cubic feet per second'.
Bendigo Advertiser, Saturday 31 January 1874, p. 2.

This walk reaches its furthest point at Fryerstown Road. For those who are doing the return walk anticlockwise, you will turn left here and then left again at Salt Water Track. For accurate navigation it's best to have a GPS device or mobile phone running a GPS app. Continue down Salt Water Track following the yellow path marked on the map (page 52). You will pass Rilen Track on your right and continue on until you reach Dearden Track where you need to turn left. At 720 m, turn right (south) on to Kemps Track. The shortcut back to the channel is about 600 metres further on (immediately after Kangaroo Creek Gully). The footpath isn't very well marked, but the channel is only 90 metres to your left (east). You can then turn right on the Channel access track and return to your starting point.

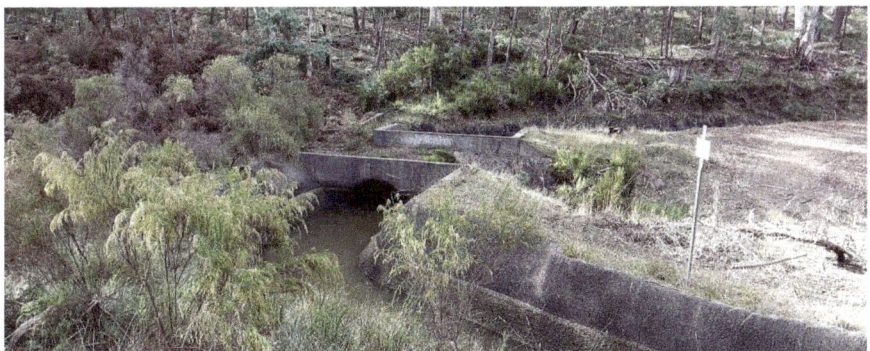

Culvert and crossover at unnamed gully, 900 metres from Dearden Track.

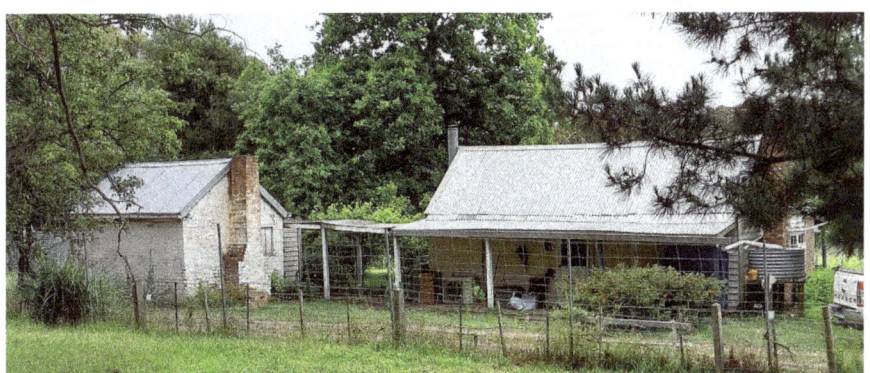

Old channel keeper's house just south of Fryerstown Road.

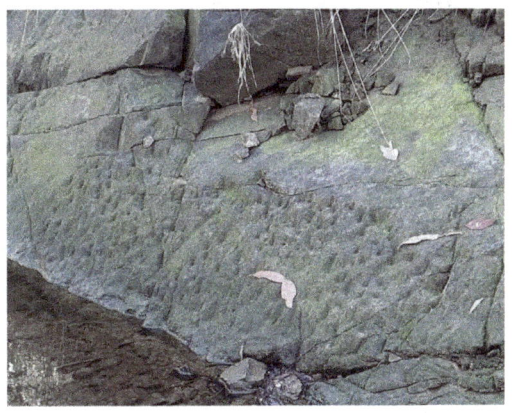

These appear to be marks made by picks during the construction of the channel.

Fryerstown Road to Wright Street, Elphinstone

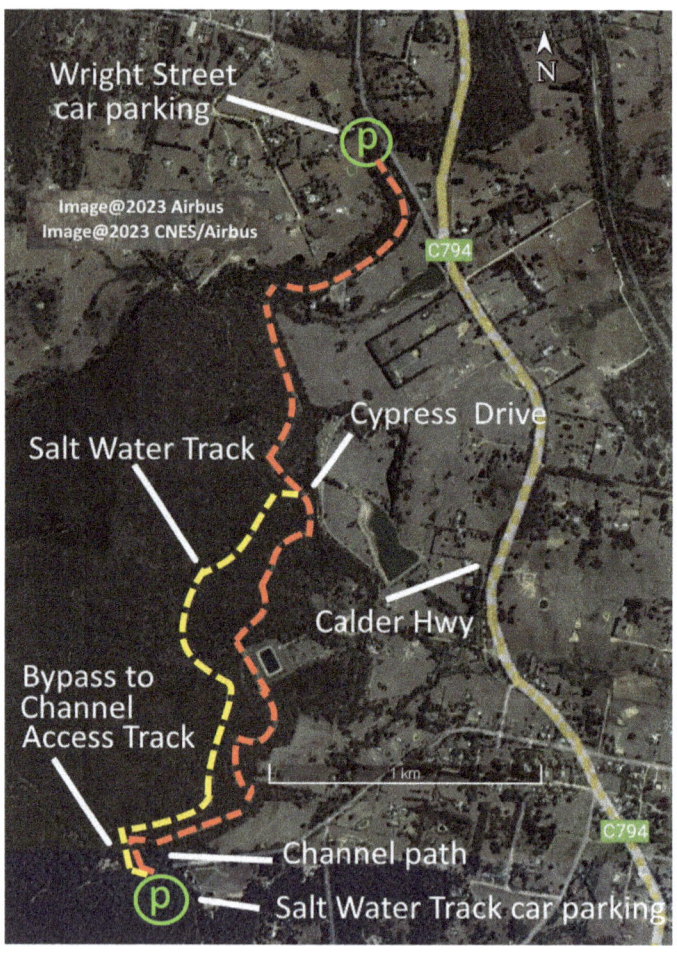

The starting point for this walk is a car parking area a little way down Salt Water Track off Fryerstown Road. If a car shuttle can be arranged, another car should be parked off the roadway at Wright Street just north of the channel crossing. Those returning to their starting point will have to backtrack some of the way from Wright Street (total distance 8 km) or else turn left at Cypress Drive and return via Salt Water Track (yellow line – 4.3 km return).

When you start at Fryerstown Road there is a choice of paths. The easiest and safest path is to avoid the channel reserve which is seldom if ever used and is overgrown. Bypass this section of the channel by walking up the continuation of Salt Water Track. About 300 metres further up the road a gate, on the right-hand side (east) leads back to the Coliban Channel access track.

While it's possible to follow the channel north from Fryerstown Road a daunting challenge faces you. The only way across to the other side of the Channel, to where the access track resumes, is along a narrow stone wall with a sheer drop on either side. Serious injury awaits anyone who tries such a feat and fails.

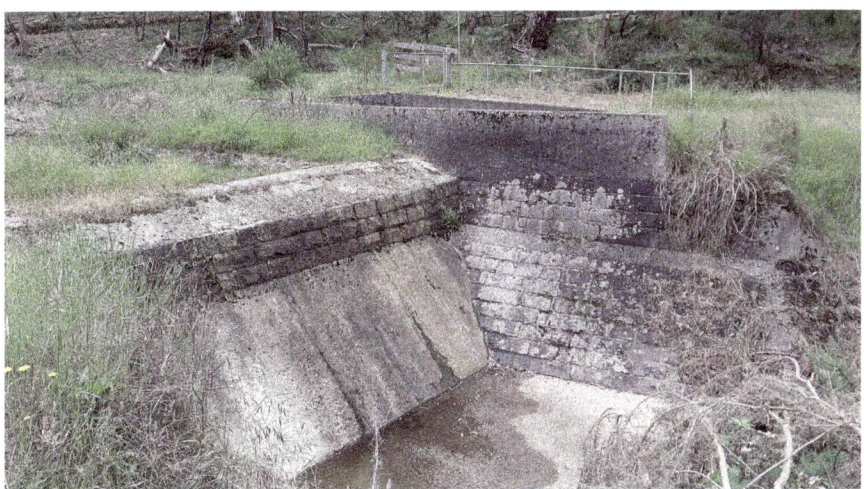

Kangaroo Creek culvert and weir.

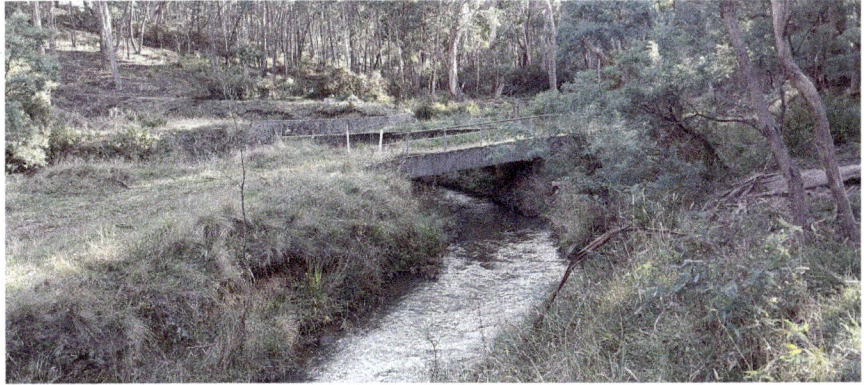

Looking back towards Kangaroo Creek culvert and crossover.

'In order to clean out the Coliban water supply channel, from Malmsbury to Castlemaine, the water was turned off on Saturday. On Sunday the channel was lined with residents, with all sorts of instruments, to harpoon the fish as the water left the channel. A large quantity was captured, among them being a trout weighing 6 lb., and another 4.5 lb. A lot of perch were also captured, the largest being 3.5 lb.'
The Age, Wednesday 4 October 1911, p. 10.

Mystery structure, perhaps a waste weir.

Along the channel there are concrete and stone structures designed to handle overflowing flood waters if the channel level should get too high during a major rain event. If the channel is allowed to overflow along a bank composed of earth, major erosion could occur which could threaten the integrity of the bank. The structure shown here may well be such a waste weir (the lack of an equivalent structure on the other higher side of the channel indicates that it wasn't an overshoot or bridge).

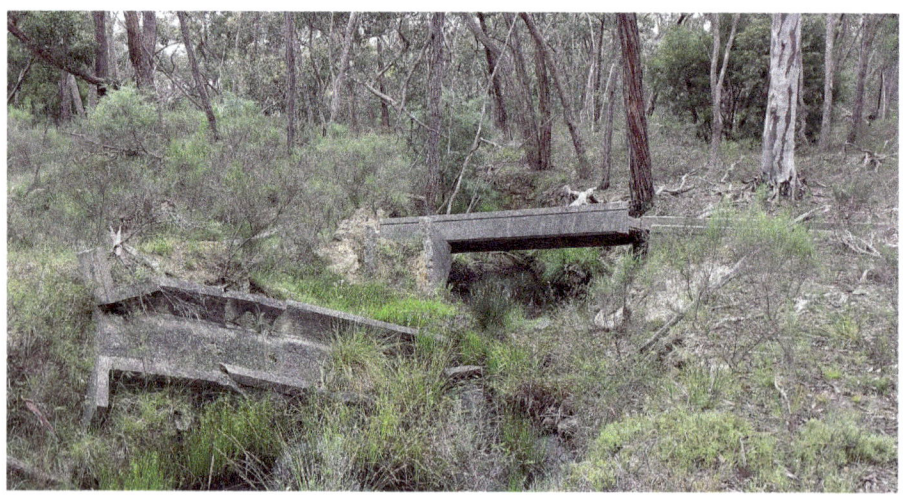

Ruined overshoots on old channel, near Cypress Drive.

At Cypress Drive, an option for those not wishing to go on to Wright Street is to turn left and return via Salt Water Track (see map). This will lead back to the starting point just south of Fryerstown Road. On the way along Cypress Drive you will cross over a section of the old decommissioned channel. It's worth having a look as it suggests how the channel might once have appeared before it was replaced by the concrete channel.

Those intending to continue on to Wright Street will soon encounter another of the deep cuttings that occur at regular intervals along the Back Creek syphon to Elphinstone section of the Coliban Channel.

> 'Between 12¼ [19.71 km] and 12½ miles [20.1 km] there is a very heavy cutting, 27 feet [8.2 m] in depth, through hard schistose-rock. The plan here has been adopted by Mr. Stone of leaving the bottom 6 feet in width instead of 4½, and carrying the sides up perpendicularly for 5 feet to a berm. By this means a great deal of excavation was avoided, and money saved, the work having been done by day labor.'
> Bendigo Advertiser, Saturday 31 January 1874, p. 2.

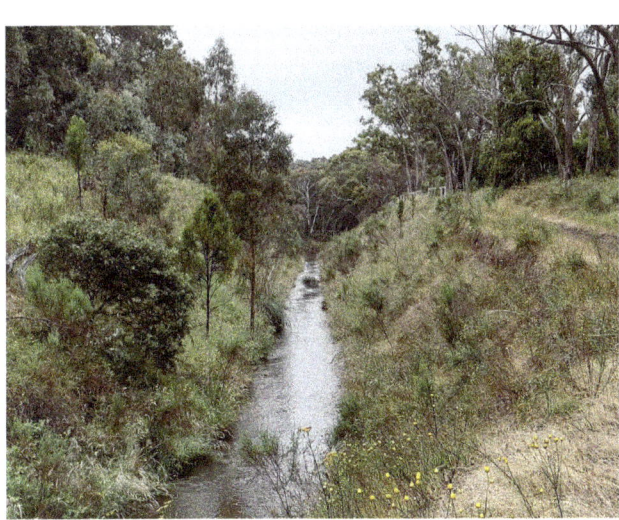
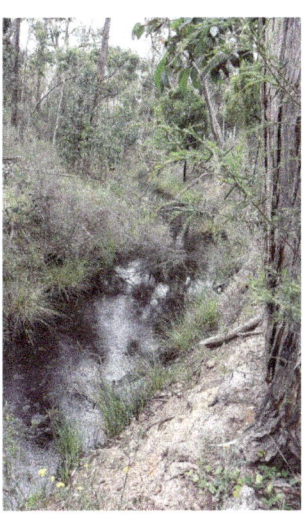

Cutting, Elphinstone.　　　　　　　　*Old bypassed channel.*

Wright Street, Elphinstone to Elphinstone township

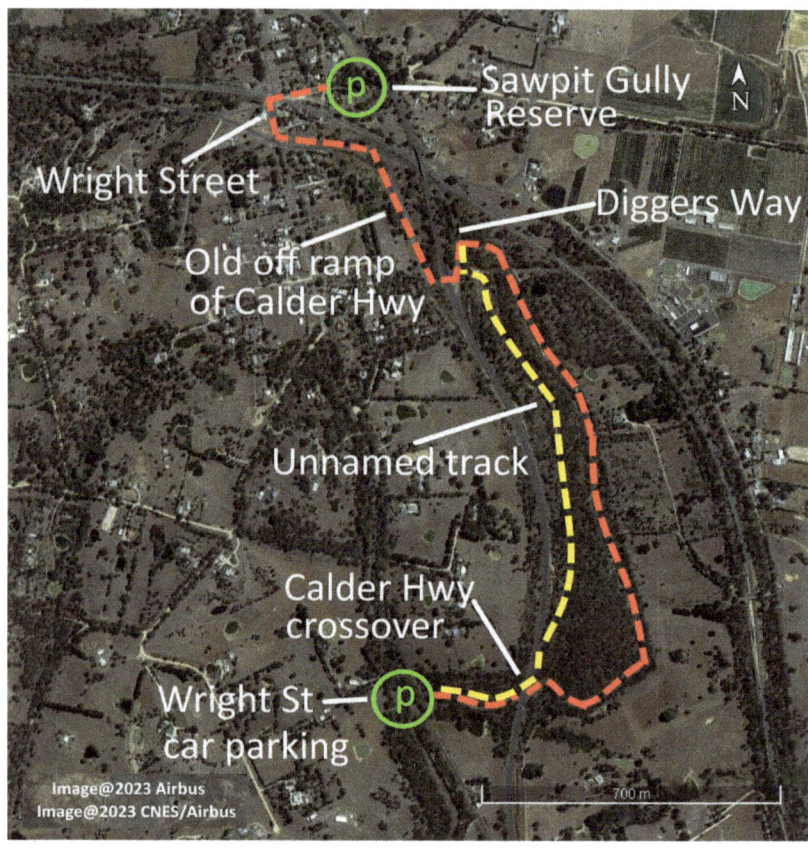

North of where the channel goes under Wright Street there is a firm grassy area on the west side suitable for car parking. A short return walk (3.5 km) begins here. Walk across the road and follow the channel. At the Calder Highway, cross over the road and continue walking along the access track for about 1.5 km. The track loops around and meets Diggers Way not far from the Elphinstone township. If you're doing the loop walk you'll turn left at Diggers Way and walk south for about 10 metres where you'll see a track running back into the forest. This well-worn track runs roughly parallel to Diggers Way and the Calder

Highway. It can be followed almost all the way back to the Calder Highway channel crossing. At this point return along the channel to your car.

> 'At 12½ miles [20.1 km] the main road [Old Melbourne Road now Wright Street] will be crossed by a culvert 58 feet [17.7 m] in length, succeeded by a flume (both let): at 12¾ miles [20.5 km] a brick level crossing (unlet). From 13 miles to 14 miles where the channel passes Elphinstone, there has been a great deal of excavation in hard schistose rock, and granite cement.'
> *Bendigo Advertiser, Saturday 31 January 1874, p. 2.*

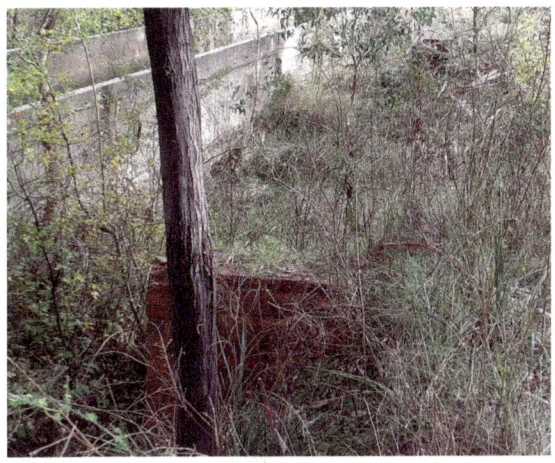

Brick piers from original flume near Wright Street.

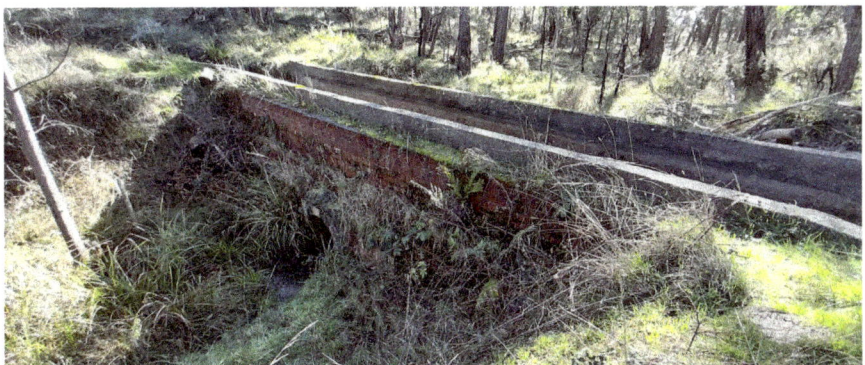

Box section brick flume, near Calder Highway Elphinstone.

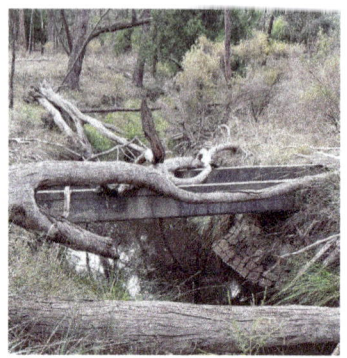 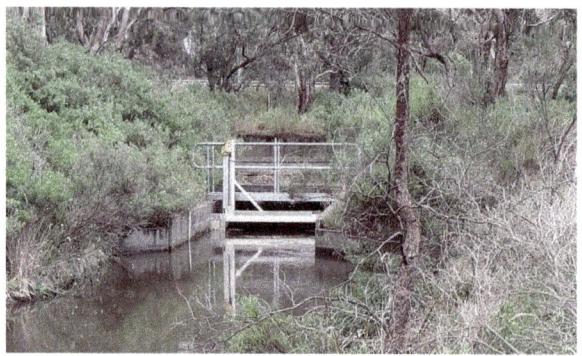

Old bypassed section of channel, Elphinstone. Right: Channel, Diggers Way.

On the other side of the Calder Highway the old 'brick level crossing' (see previous page) has been adapted to incorporate a new section of concrete flume.

Those who have combined multiple walks or are simply completing their car shuttle walk might now prefer to simply take a short cut by crossing over to an old bypassed off ramp of the Calder Highway (having to climb over yet another gate!) and then proceed on to Wright Street. Walk past the Elphinstone Hotel (where, with luck, a refreshing ale might be available!) and over the railway crossing before turning into Urquhart Street and heading to Sawpit Gully Reserve, corner of Urquhart and Doveton Streets (refer map page 64). Here, besides a car parking area, there are toilets, a shelter with electric BBQs, a phone box, and a power outlet (although this might not be permanently available). Next to the reserve is a post office/general store which is open weekdays, and weekend mornings.

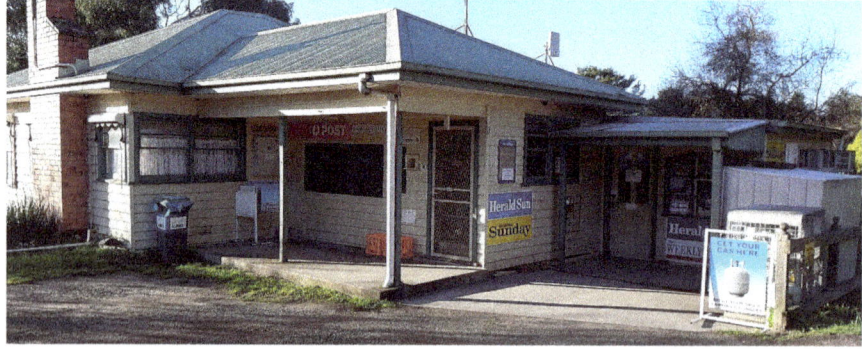

Elphinstone Post Office/General Store, Doveton Street.

Apparently, not long ago, camping was allowed in the park here but it became overly popular when someone listed the spot in a Free Camping book and the privilege was withdrawn. It's a shame because it would be a perfect place for hikers to spend the night. Nevertheless, the nearby Fryers Ranges offer many opportunities for informal camping. One example is the Oven Rock Campground, Fryers Ridge Track.

Those not wanting to detour but to follow the channel through the back streets of this side of Elphinstone will find the going far from easy. In fact, it's more trouble than it's worth. Not only is there some uncertainty as to whether the channel actually runs through freehold land, one short section is overgrown with blackberry and gorse and is difficult to access.

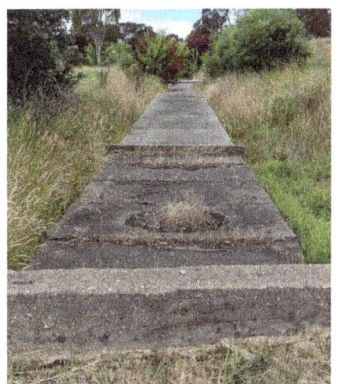
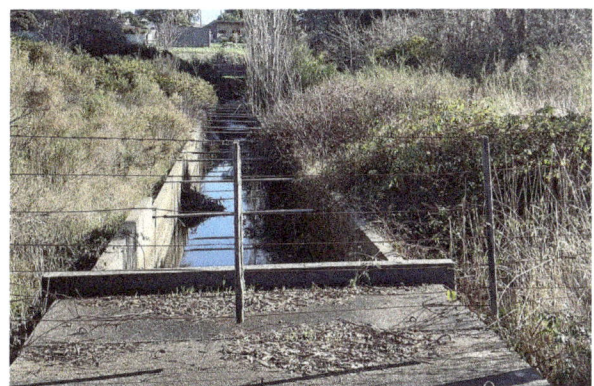

Some features of the channel between the Calder Highway and Wright Street.

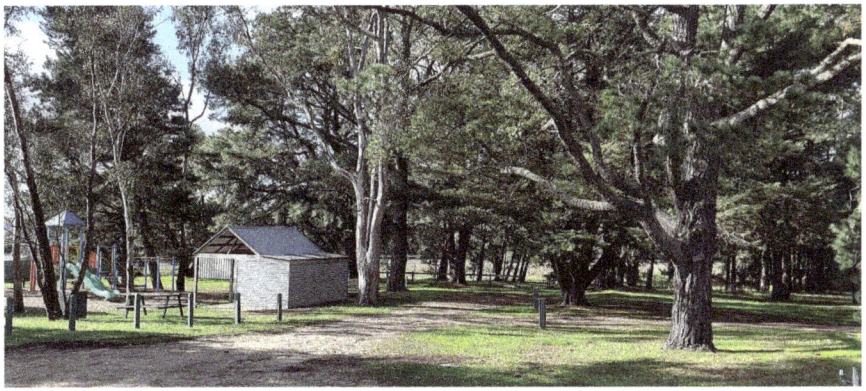

Sawpit Gully Reserve, Urquhart Street.

The Channel at Elphinstone

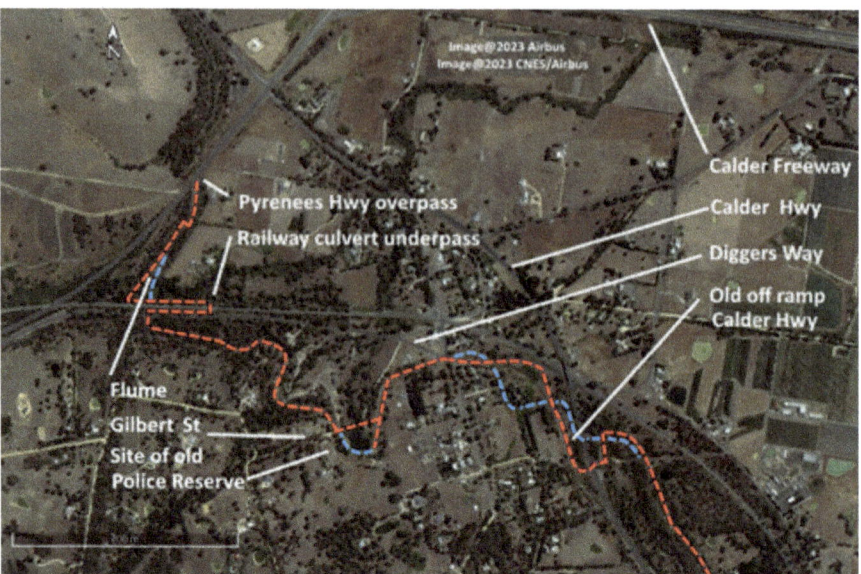

Most of the channel within the Elphinstone township is either within freehold land, not navigable or has prohibited entry. About the only stretch of the channel which is easily accessible is between Wright Street and Gilbert Street. It's possible to walk the channel between Gilbert Street and Diggers Way, but for some reason there is a sign on the Gilbert Street access track gate which has a Do Not Enter sign, even though anyone walking in from Diggers Way faces no similar sign.

However, for those wishing to know what the channel looks like as it meanders through Elphinstone, the following description is provided. I'll begin at the point reached in the previous walk. The red hatched line is the path I took, and the blue hatched line is the line of the channel itself and marks where our paths diverged.

At Diggers Way there is a culvert that carries the channel under the road. When it emerges on the other side, it is covered in concrete slabs (to prevent polluted material entering the channel). There is another culvert under the Calder Highway, and on the other side, the channel is again mostly hidden under concrete except for a small section of open channel near the Doveton Street extension (see photos page 67).

At the intersection of Wright Street and Diggers Way the channel crosses diagonally beneath the intersection and surfaces within the gated Coliban Water Reserve. This is the short accessible section mentioned above.

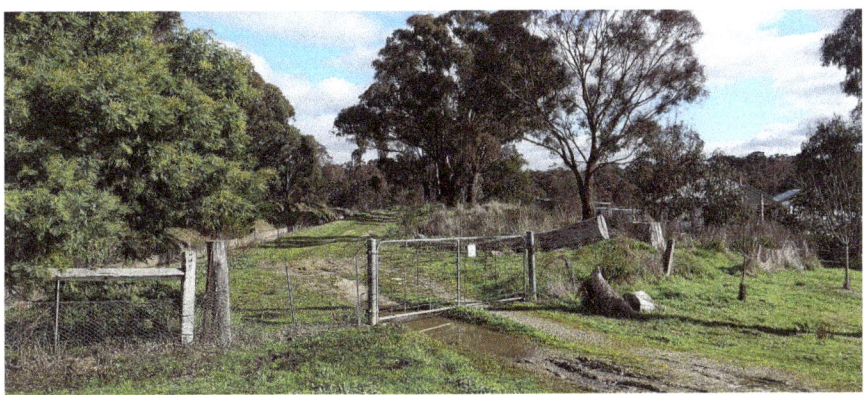

Gate near Diggers Way, Wright Street intersection.

You will need to step over the barbed wire fence next to the gate to follow the channel.

At the end of the track there is yet another trash grate and a sluice (below) which allows water to be diverted from the channel into a tributary of Sawpit Gully. But that's about as far as you can go because the channel swings to the west over an overgrown creek. Although there isn't a NO ENTRY sign facing you here, if you manage to get past the gully you will learn you shouldn't have entered this area by the sign on the gate at Gilbert Street.

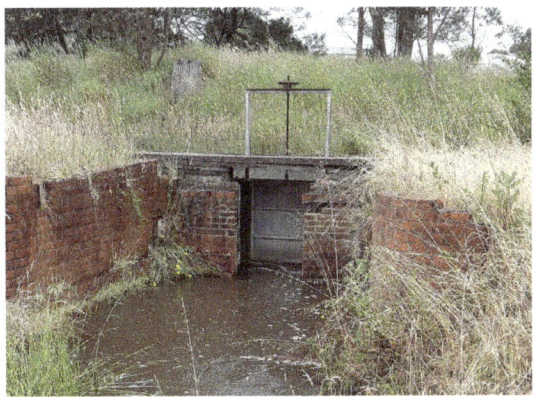

Sluice near Old Police Paddock Elphinstone.

At Gilbert Street, not only is there a NO ENTRY: AUTHORISED PERSONS ONLY sign behind you on the east access track gate, but there's also one on the west gate facing you. It's by no means obvious why public access is prohibited here.

> 'From the Elphinstone police paddock,[26] the aqueduct line runs along at the back of the Episcopalian Church[27] up to the main road and railway crossing. ... At the point where the aqueduct intersects the main road and railway at Elphinstone, the rail and road run parallel with each other; consequently, to carry the aqueduct across this point will be a delicate, if not difficult, operation, as the railway embankment will have to be cut into ...'
> Leader, Saturday 31 January 1874, p. 20.

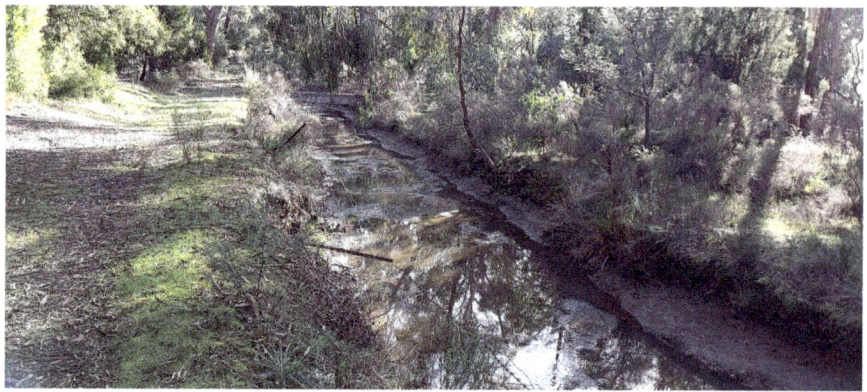

Channel access track between Gilbert Street and Diggers Way.

By the time Diggers Way is reached the access track has narrowed to a walking track. A culvert carries the channel beneath both Diggers Way (the old Pyrenees Highway) and the railway line embankment.

Bushwalkers who walk for fun rather than adventure should probably give Elphinstone a miss and head straight to the Sutton Grange section, but here's a description of the channel north of the railway line for those who are curious. Looking at the map it might appear that if you want to follow the channel all you need

---

26 The Elphinstone Police Paddock was located in Gilbert Street next to the Main Channel. Later, it was the location of the Elphinstone water bailiff.

27 Now a privately owned reception centre.

do is cross over the railway line. However, even apart from the safety concerns, this is impossible as there's a three metre high wire fence on the other side of the line. In my case, I had to go *under* the railway line.

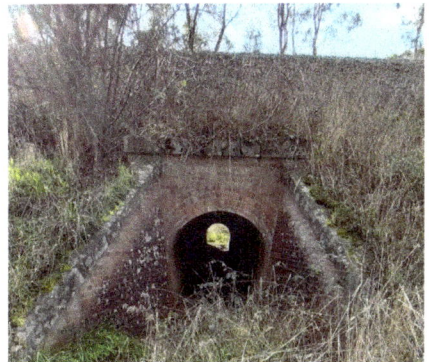 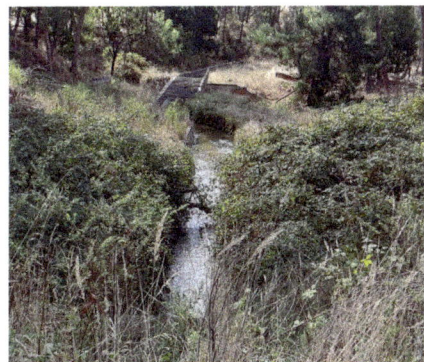

Culvert leading to a blackberry infested wilderness. Right: View of channel from railway embankment.

Luckily there's a culvert in the railway embankment some distance along Diggers Way. It's large enough to walk through. On the other side there's a daunting thicket of blackberries. However I found a path of sorts leading off left along the base of the embankment. Faced with a mountain of blackberries, I climbed up the embankment (there is something of a sloping path) and found that at the top there was enough room to walk along next to the fence until I made it past the channel below me.

I carefully made my way down through the trees to the channel trying to avoid the blackberries which have a nasty habit of catching on clothes and skin. This was once a delightful picnic spot, with an ornate brick channel culvert and flume (see photo next page).

It's no easy task crossing the blackberry-choked gully, but once I'd done that I walked along the west side of the channel until I could cross over to the access track via a concrete overshoot 200 metres further on.

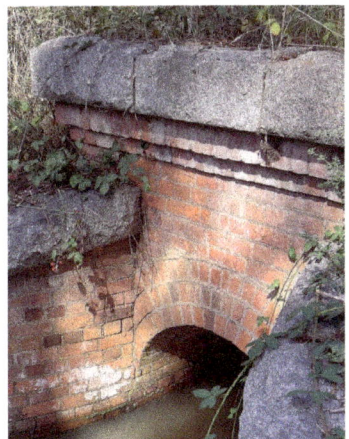

Close up of railway line culvert outlet.

The concrete race becomes an open channel at the point where it cuts through a stony ridge. The only thing detracting from the pretty sight is the infestation of tree lucerne growing along the channel. Farmers don't seem to mind this weedy tree, but it took me many years to control its spread on my bush block. I'll continue the description of the channel beyond the Pyrenees Highway overpass in the next section, which is also equally challenging.

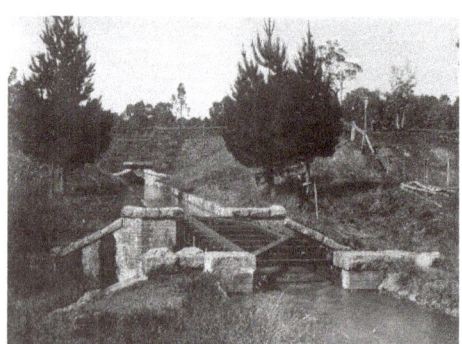 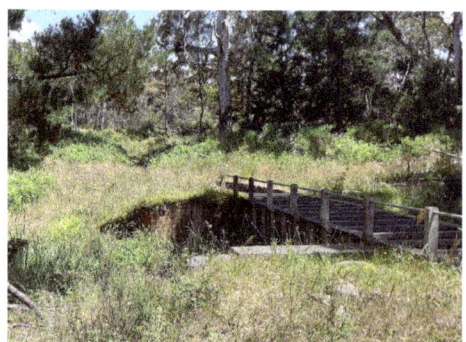

Railway line culvert outlet and flume, 1940, SR&WSC. Right: The same location today, looking south towards Railway embankment.[28]

'A system for the purpose of irrigating land situated above the water channel has just been installed here (writes our Elphinstone correspondent), and its success is practically assured. It means a big thing, to this and adjoining districts, as there is a lot of splendid land above the water channels lying practically idle, owing to there being no cheap and effective system of irrigating it. This difficulty has apparently now been solved, as is now being demonstrated by Mr. J. H. Timmins of this locality.

Mr. Timmins' residence, "The Glen," is situated alongside the main Melbourne road, and about 500 yards above the Coliban channel. Recently he opened up negotiations with Mr. C. Beer, of Boort, for the supply and erection of a windmill for irrigation purposes .... It is built about 50ft from the water race ... The water runs into the tank and through 1-inch pipes, a distance of about 200 yards to the highest point where a stand pipe is

---

28 The original timber flume has been replaced by a concrete flume and displaced from the original line. Stonework is now hidden by grass and weeds.

erected 70ft above the level of the water channel. There are five taps— one in the kitchen, one at the horse trough, one at the dairy, and two in the garden, and at each the pressure is splendid. His is now one of the most comfortable homesteads in the district, and other residents on the high side of the race will doubtless soon follow his splendid example'
Mount Alexander Mail, Tuesday 25 February 1913, p. 2.

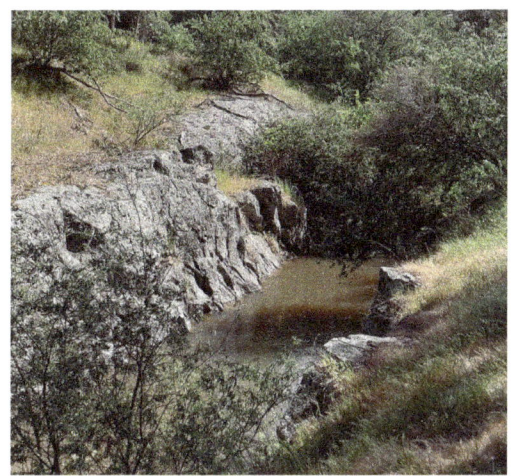

The channel leading up to Pyrenees Highway overpass.

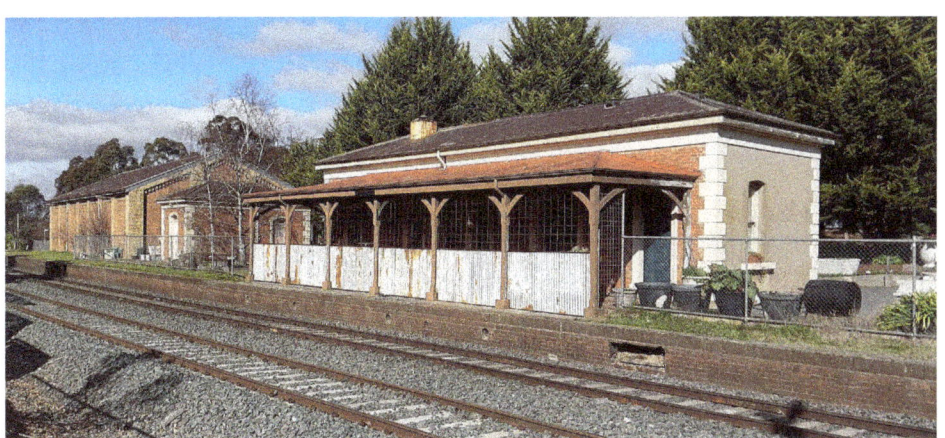

The disused Elphinstone railway station.

Elphinstone to Ellerys Road, Faraday

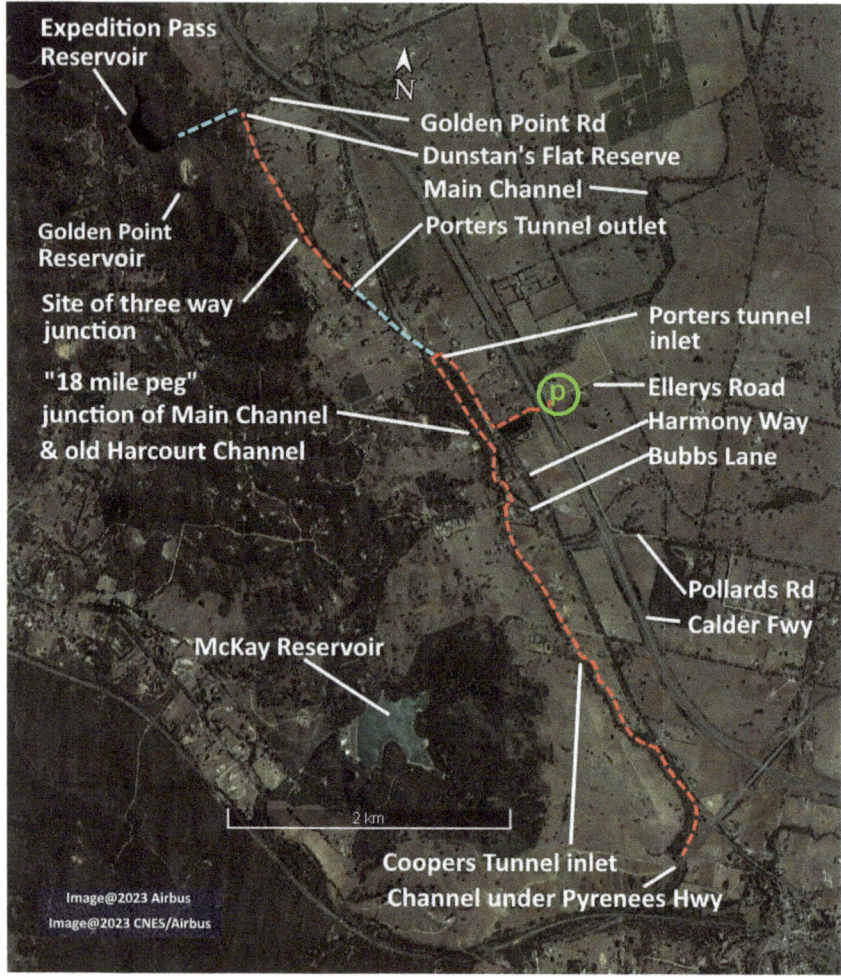

The same advice applies to this section of the channel as to the previous Elphinstone section. The access track is intermittent here and mostly not maintained. Within the Coliban Channel reserve, rank grass and weeds of every description make good hiding places for snakes, and near the junction of the Main Channel and the old Harcourt Channel and the Coliban Pumping Station, there is some uncertainty as to permission of access. Between Porters

Tunnel and Golden Point Road, the channel runs through freehold land, and even if access was granted, there's no track of any kind.

Nevertheless, the following is a description of the channel in this section. The blue dashed line represents the underground path of Porters Tunnel and of the creek flowing into Expedition Pass Reservoir.

The Pyrenees Highway overpass was reached in the last section. Near the overpass the channel disappears under a protective cloak of concrete panels. The panels make for easy walking, but the blackberries have no trouble finding a toehold.

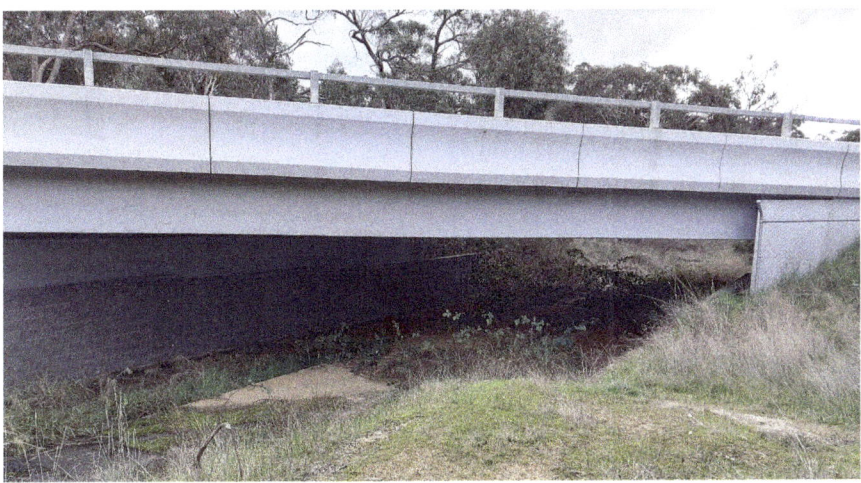

Pyrenees Highway overpass.

Once through the underpass, care needs to be exercised because one slab has a panel missing. Apparently, in the 1870s, there was a road and a crossing over the channel near this location.

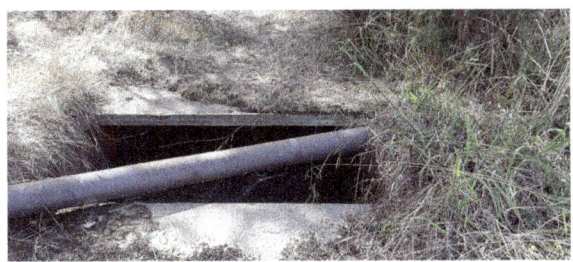

Not the time to be looking down at your phone!

'At sixteen miles fifteen chains [26.05 km] a place known as the Occupation Road crossing is a rough log [bridge] made over the aqueduct. It is so rough that no dray could safely cross it, and so clumsy that water could not pass freely under it.'
The Age, Thursday 29 January 1874, p. 3.

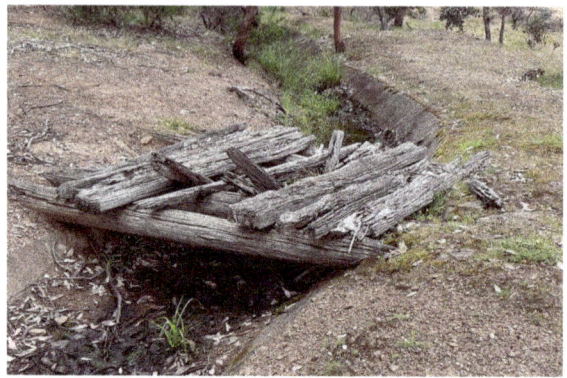

The occasional 'rough log bridge' still survives, this one on the Golden Point Reservoir channel.

The access track runs parallel to and close to Harmony Way, but it soon swings away to meet the road. A rough foot track continues along the channel, and just when you start to think it's becoming impassable, the access track re-enters the Coliban Channel reserve from the road.

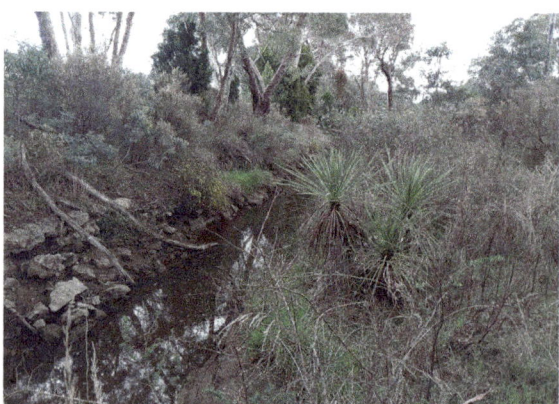

Channel near Harmony Way.

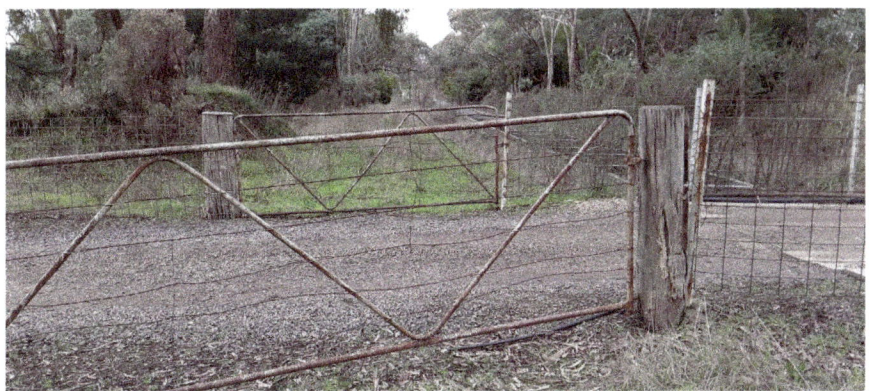
Access track gates near Harmony Way, Faraday, looking south.

Further along, a bridge and a fenced track allow a farmer to access land on either side of the channel.

Stretches of the old bypassed channel, here and elsewhere, have great beauty and are important flora and fauna refuges in an otherwise greatly altered landscape.

At almost two kilometres from the Pyrenees Highway, the side channel to Coopers Tunnel is reached. This allows water to be

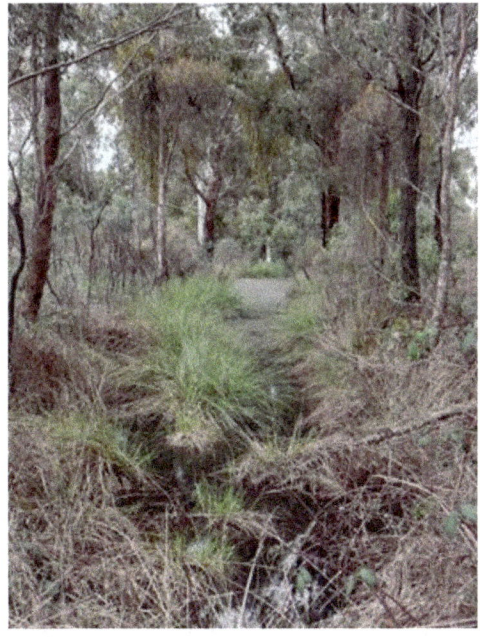
A bypassed channel, Faraday.

diverted to McCay Reservoir on the other side of the ridge. From there, the Poverty Gully race once conveyed water to Norwood Hill in Castlemaine and to Crocodile Reservoir, Fryerstown. The Poverty Gully race, although narrower than the Main channel, is itself an extraordinary feat of engineering. Much of its length can be walked and there are still many historic features along it.

On the other side of the ridge, the outlet of Coopers Tunnel meets a short length of open channel that leads to a small reservoir built in 1874 (just above the much more recent McCay Reservoir). From here the old Poverty Gully race leads to a syphon which once conveyed water under the railway line to emerge in the Fryers Ranges where the open channel resumes. Two tunnels and an interesting series of stone waterfalls near Fryerstown Road are among the many historic features that have survived to the present day.

> 'It is intended to furnish a sufficient supply for mining purposes to the gold workers at Castlemaine, Chewton, and Fryerstown, by means of an open race, and a tunnel [Coopers Tunnel], of a minimum height of 6ft. and a width of 4ft., is now being driven from a point on the main channel 17 miles [27.4 km] from Malmsbury for a distance of above half a mile to conduct the water into the race ... When this is completed, the miners will be able to obtain a supply of 5,000,000gal. a day direct from the Malmsbury reservoir, and the main from Expedition Pass will then be used only for the domestic supply.' The
> *Argus, Saturday 7 August 1875, p. 4.*

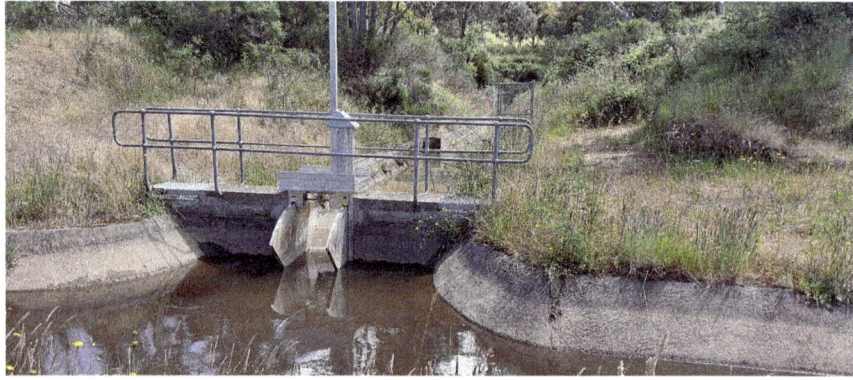

Junction showing channel leading to Coopers Tunnel (and McCay Reservoir).

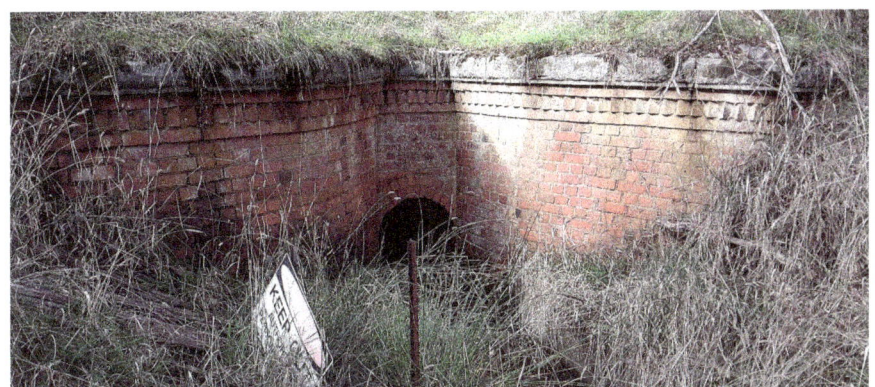

Coopers Tunnel outlet, McCay Reservoir.

From the Coopers Tunnel channel it's only a short distance to Old Chapel Lane which makes me think there was an old church building here at one stage. This provides access to Harmony Way (the old Melbourne Road). One kilometre later, Bubbs Lane is reached. To the west, not far from the channel, are the stone ruins of a house owned by the farmer who gave his name to this Lane.

> 'At the second bridge [Bubbs Lane] on the Malmsbury side of Porter's tunnel, a man[29] has recovered from the Government

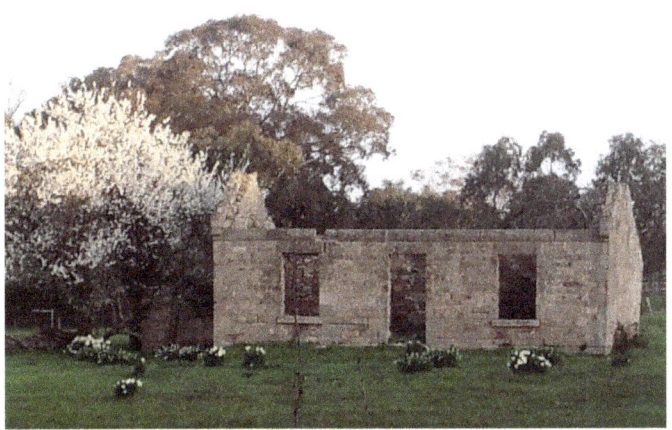

Bubbs cottage, Bubbs Lane, Faraday.

---

29 Almost certainly Isaac Bubb whose house and property bordered the channel here. The ruins of his 1860s era granite house are a local landmark in Bubbs Lane (once known as Bubb's Road).

three different sums as compensation, to which he was justly entitled, for damage done to his land, owing to the uncompleted state of the works and in all probability he will get a fourth when the next flood comes down.'
The Age, Thursday 29 January 1874, p. 3.

The access track on the north side of Bubbs Lane appears to be rarely used. However, there's a lovely rural feel to the channel here, and the native birdlife is especially prolific in this section leading to Porters Tunnel. Sacred kingfishers, woodswallows, quite a few different honeyeater species, as well as some less common birds can be regularly observed here.

In approximately 400 metres the 18 mile peg is reached. Even early on it was recognized that the distance from Malmsbury to this point was slightly less than 18 miles (owing to some changes made to the proposed course of the channel before excavation was started), but the name stuck.

> 'At the old 18-mile peg (now 17¾ miles) the height of the bottom of the channel above sea level is 1,360½ feet, and at the point of divergence a large tank has been built of brick, with

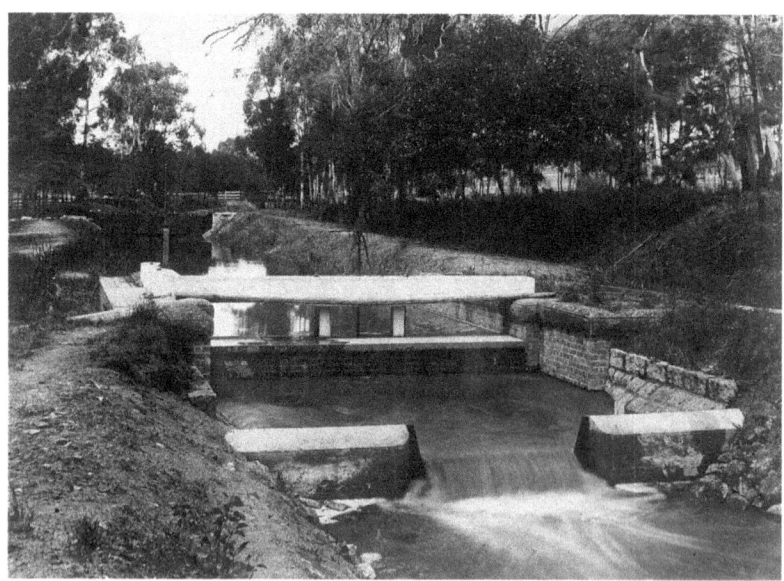

The original junction tank and sluices, 1900.

handsome bluestone copings, solid massive granite wings and aprons and cast iron sluice gates (to Castlemaine and Sandhurst respectively) strengthened by very strong beams of best Sydney ironbark, specially picked for the purpose, as there is a particular strain at this point. The internal dimensions of the tank are 18 feet x 10 feet, and the sluices are so arranged that a simultaneous supply of water can be sent along both channels or either one of them as desired.'
Bendigo Advertiser, Tuesday 20 November 1877, p. 2.

'At the eighteen-mile peg there is a ... tank being fitted with sluice gates across the main channel, one branch of which runs to Castlemaine[30] and the other to Sandhurst. These gates can be used in any manner circumstances may demand. The water can be let down both channels simultaneously, or one or other of the two, as the case may require. ... It should be here explained that a very clever device has been hit upon in the construction of the culverts, syphons and flumes along the whole line. The inclination of their dip has in all cases been materially increased, as compared to the declension of the main channel, so as to accelerate the flow, and thereby make their carrying capacity large in comparison to the breadth and depth of the conduit.'
The Age Thursday 3 January 1878 p. 3.

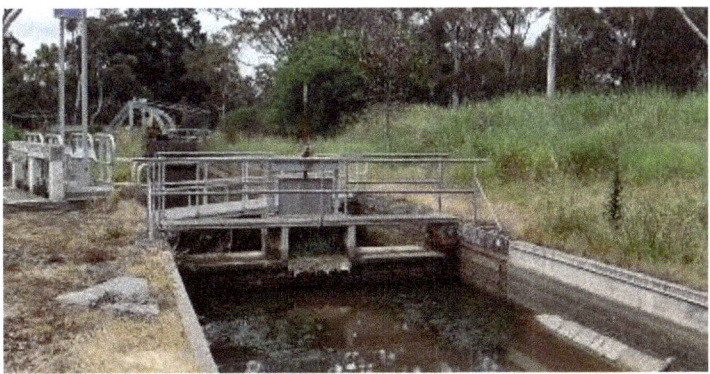

Present day view of the original junction tank.

---

30 Remember that the channel was originally designed to supply Castlemaine with water from a pipe coming from the Expedition Pass Reservoir.

I'll describe the old Expedition Pass Reservoir channel and then return to the junction to continue along the Coliban Main Channel. Within about 300 metres from the channel junction there is a deep cutting which ends in about 800 metres at the No. 2 (Porters) Tunnel, near Kennedys Lane.

> 'Passing under a rough wooden bridge the branch channel continues in a straight line with the main, of which it is rather a continuation than a branch, towards Expedition Pass reservoir, the entire distance being 1 mile 66 chains [2.9 km]. The portion of the channel approaching tunnel No. 2 [Porters] Tunnel is well cut, and with the exception of one rather extensive slip on the lower side, appears to be in an excellent state of preservation. For some [distance] there is a very deep cutting, the upper portion of which and all above the tunnel entrance is beautifully turfed, this work having been done many years ago, in Mr. Christopherson's time. It has stood well, and will bear favorable comparison with any work of a similar description in the colony.
>
> I may mention that on the slope, about half-way between the entrance and the crown of the embankment, there is a magnificent spring of cool water, welling up from the granite formation. It is easily reached, and to the thirsty traveller on a hot summer's day affords a most welcome relief.'
> *Bendigo Advertiser, 4 February 1874, p. 2.*

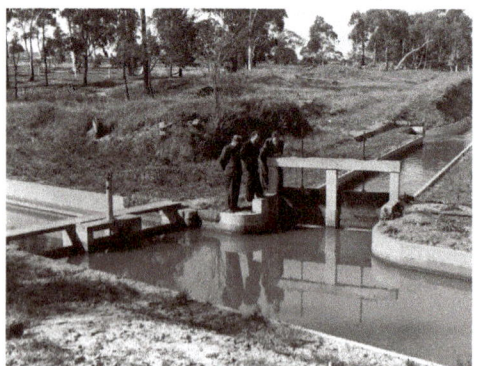 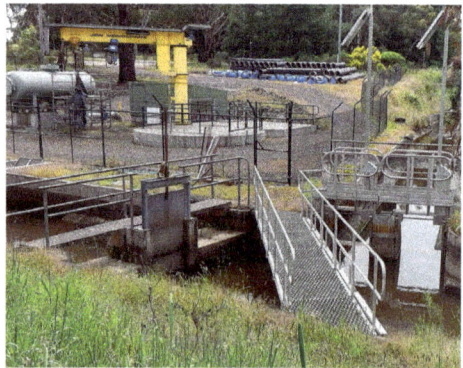

Junction of channels looking east. Old Harcourt channel on left, 1946 SR&WSC. Right: Same location, 2022.

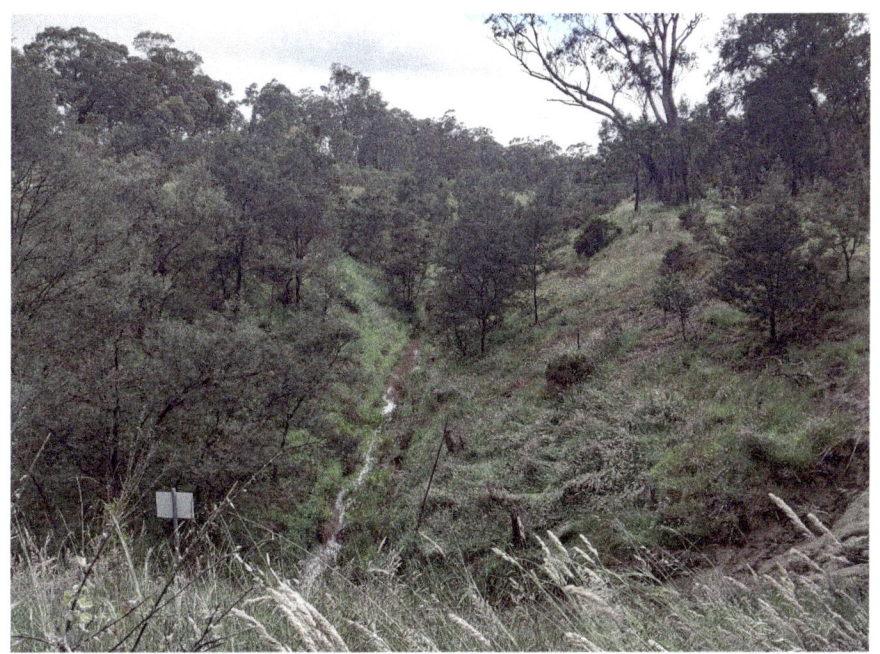

Cutting near No. 2 (Porters) Tunnel.

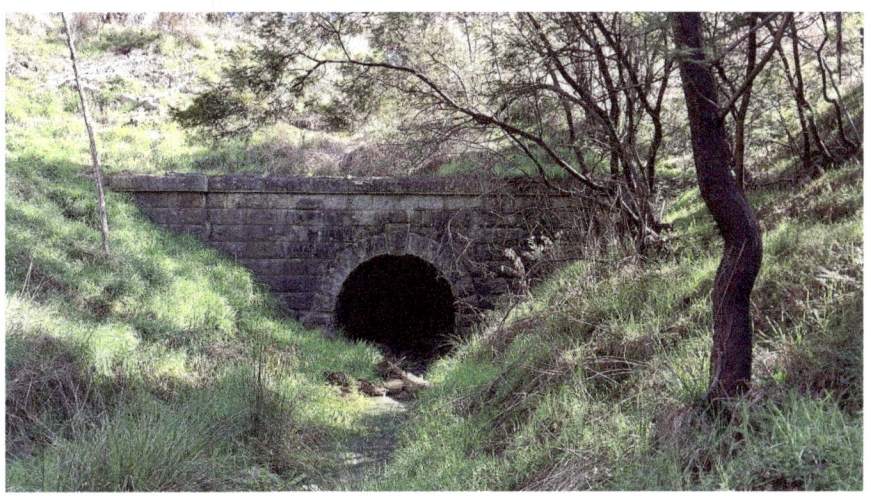

No. 2 (Porters) Tunnel entrance.

Porters Tunnel to Expedition Pass Reservoir

'Throughout its [Porters Tunnel] length there are several circular brick-lined air shafts, surmounted by parapets with heavy, dressed granite cope-stones. This section of the work certainly appears to have been done in an extravagant style of ornamentation, considering that it is many miles in the bush. In fact here as elsewhere, along the works, although Mr. Christopherson has not neglected the utilitarian, he seems to have allowed his love for the aesthetic to get the better of what should have been a judicious exercise of economy. The work altogether is a most substantial one, as unquestionably it ought to be for the money'
Bendigo Advertiser, 4 February 1874, p. 2.

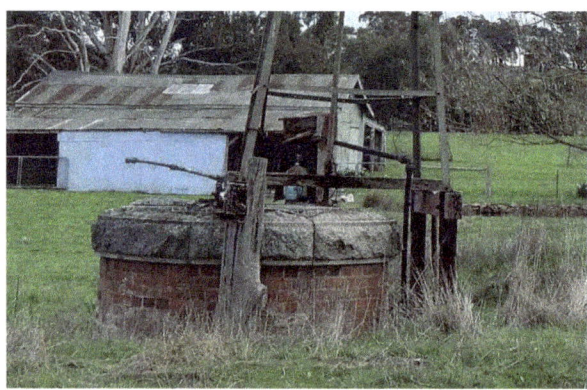

Circular brick-lined air shaft (and windmill ruins).

'An inspection of the Expedition Pass Watershed affords conclusive proof that the water which runs through it will never be fit for domestic purposes. It is intersected by several roads, the dirt and dust from which all run into the reservoir. When Porter's tunnel was opened into this watershed, the stream it brought down was turned, unrestricted, into the natural water channel. This augmentation of the natural stream, acting on a rotten granite formation at a very steep gradient, has had the

effect of tearing up the ground in a most terrific manner. The silt, as a matter of course, runs down into the reservoir, which is being filled up at an astounding rate.'
Leader, Saturday 31 January 1874, p. 20.

'Leaving the reservoir, I proceeded along the part of the channel which supplies it with water from Malmsbury to the point of divergence of the Sandhurst branch. In forming this channel advantage has been taken of a natural gully or creek, along which the water is led, falling over a number of weirs, lately completed, which break the rush of the water, and prevent silt from being scoured into the reservoir.'
Bendigo Advertiser, Tuesday 20 November 1877, p. 2.

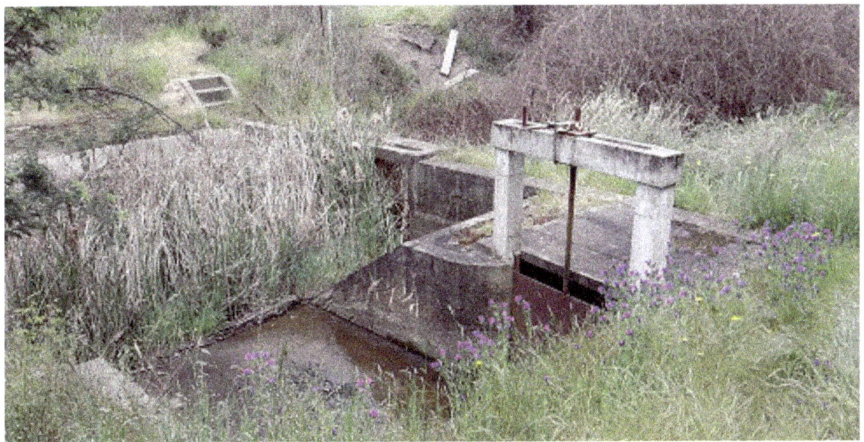

Sluice gates on Expedition Pass channel. The channel once split three ways here, the left-hand channel to the Golden Point Reservoir, the middle (the natural stream bed) to Expedition Pass Reservoir and on the right, the Harcourt Channel.

'... About half way-down the west side of the creek channel, 1 mile 24 chains [1.6 km] from where the branch diverges, there was pointed out to me the spot where, had the Coliban Scheme been carried out in its integrity, [sic] another branch would have diverged. It was originally intended that here the Castlemaine district branch should divide into two branches, one to supply the goldfields south of Forest Creek, and the other, the Harcourt branch, 11 miles in length, to terminate at the Barker's Creek Reservoir. The South Forest Creek aqueduct

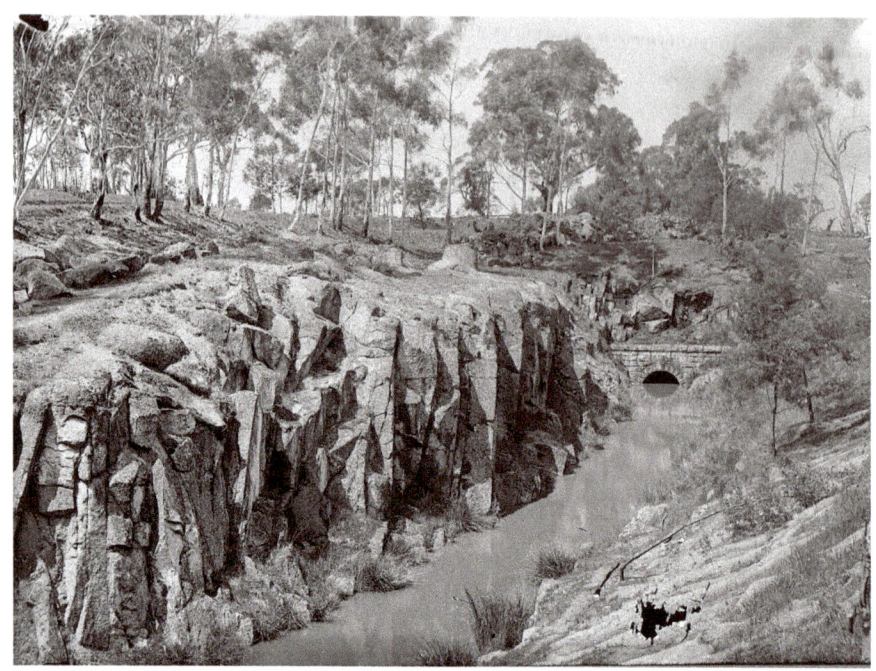

No. 2 (Porters) Tunnel outlet.

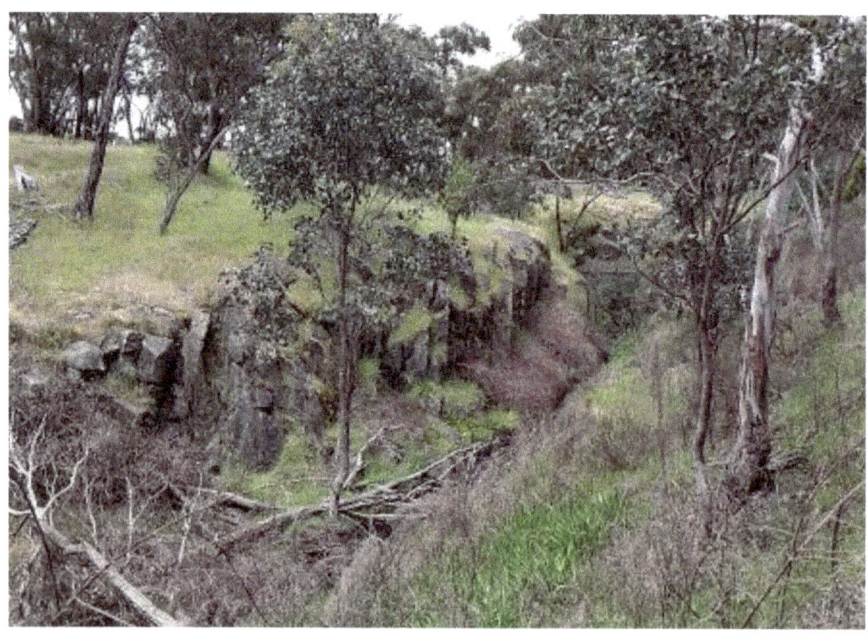

Present day view of the above location.

was to have two branches ; one to the east for the supply of the Fryerstown district, and one to the west to supply the country to the east of Campbell's Creek. It was also intended to be connected with the Expedition Pass Reservoir. The Harcourt aqueduct, it was proposed, should have two branches to supply the goldfields to the east of Barker's Creek and to the north of Forest Creek.'
Bendigo Advertiser, 4 February 1874, p. 2.

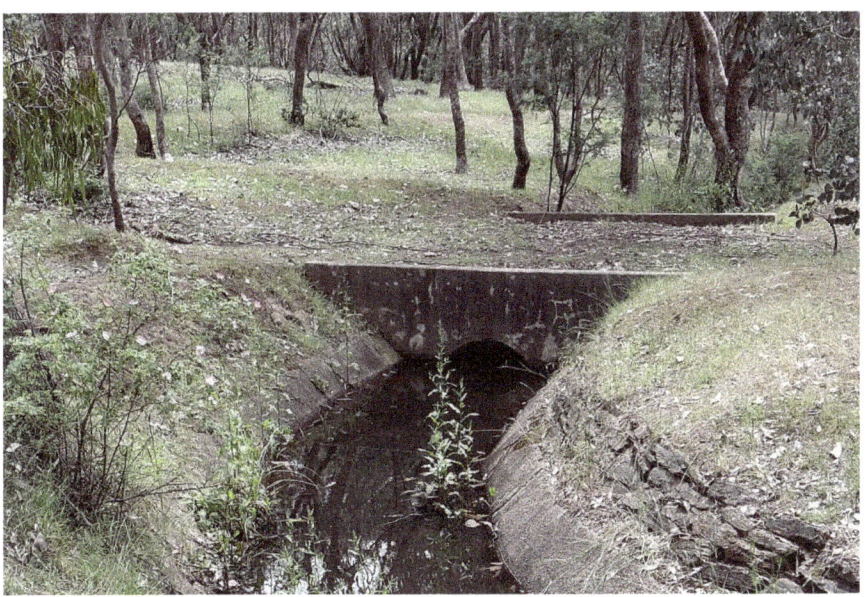

A bridge on the Golden Point Reservoir channel.

'In this gully I counted 24 of these weirs each 20 feet [6.1 m] wide across the stream by various depths, averaging about 10 feet, and very strongly built of granite. The taking advantage of this natural channel must have made a great saving in the cost of this portion of the work, and, so far as I could ascertain, fulfilled the object in view as well as could be wished, the slopes on each side have been trimmed, and are well grassed, the reserve of ground fenced with wire and top rail, and where roads intersect, strong bridges erected, and handsome gates hung at the crossings.'
The Bendigo Advertiser, 20 November 1877, p. 2.

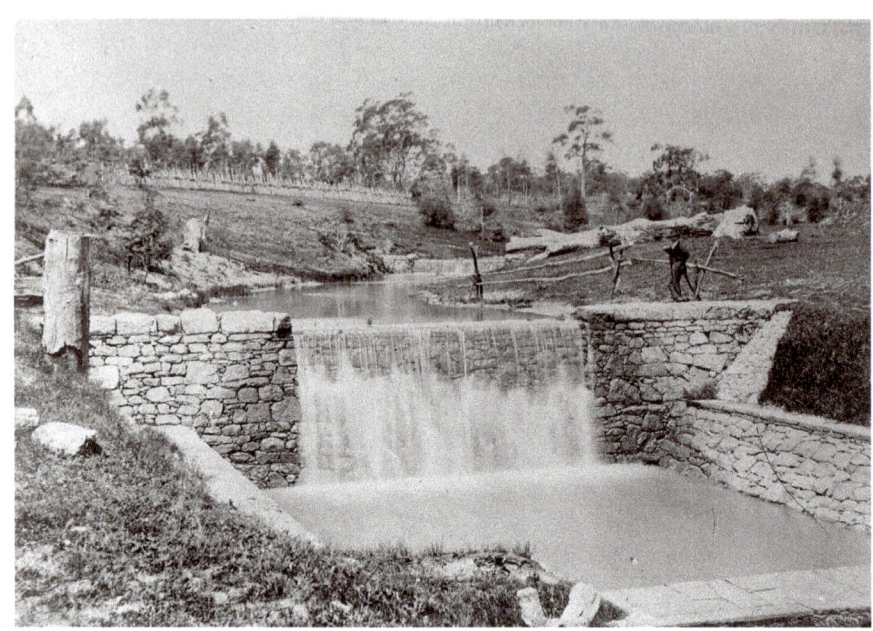

Expedition Pass channel, bottom weir.

'After visiting [some] sluicing claims I went along the road to the Expedition Pass Reservoir, and on sighting the embankment was struck by its apparent insignificance. This feeling, however, gave way to one of admiration on reaching the top as it became clear that the smallness of the bank had nothing to do with the holding capacity of the reservoir, and it struck me as being the best natural site for a work of this description that could possibly have been chosen in this locality. The Expedition Pass Reservoir is now simply a service reservoir connected with the Malmsbury Reservoir by an open channel of about 19 miles [30.58 km] in length ... It supplies the towns of Chewton, Castlemaine, and Campbell's Creek by a 12-inch main reducing to six

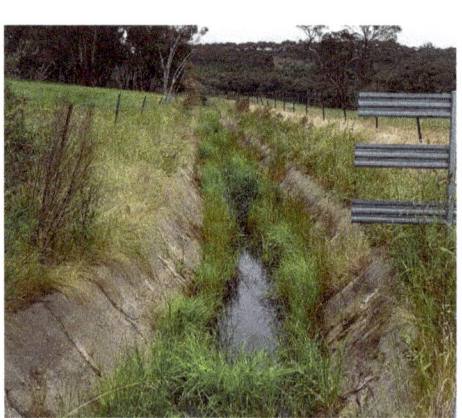

Old Harcourt channel near Expedition Pass.

inches, which affords an ample and abundant supply to them for all purposes...'.
Bendigo Advertiser, Tuesday 20 November 1877, p. 2.

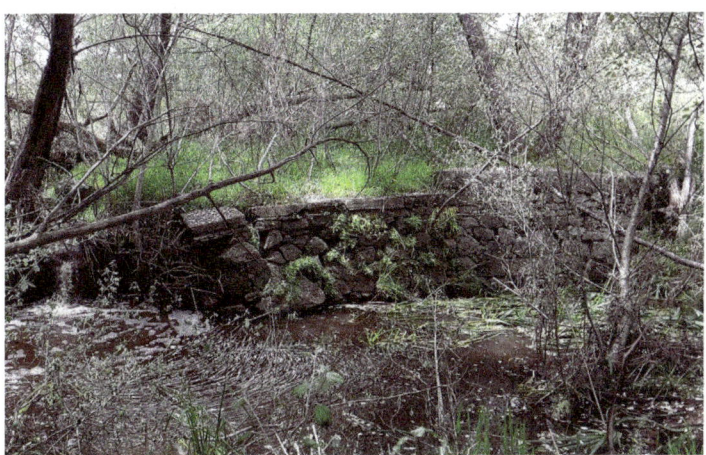

Expedition Pass channel, bottom weir, present day view.

This article from the *Mount Alexander Mail,* April 11 1913, suggests that the small, now almost forgotten, Golden Point Reservoir was constructed to improve the quality of water Castlemaine was receiving. Another benefit of the new reservoir was its higher elevation which, it was thought, would improve the water pressure in the more elevated parts of Castlemaine, much for the same reasons the Big Hill High Level Reservoir was constructed (see page 197). Once McCay Reservoir was built in 1960 there was no longer a need for this reservoir.

FARADAY.

Castlemaine townspeople will be interested to learn that a start has been made towards securing a purer water supply for the town. On Tuesday last an official of the Water Supply Department chose a site for a new reservoir near the Golden Point rifle range, not far from the present reservoir. On Wednesday morning surveyors were at work making the necessary surveys. The channel to be constructed will tap the Coliban water channel above the Expedition Pass falls, come round the hills on the south side of the road, and carry water direct to the new reservoir. Under the scheme the drainage from the majority of houses in Faraday, which at present finds its way into the town water supply, will be excluded. The present reservoir will probably be kept for the use of sluicers.

Time to return to the old 18 mile peg and resume my description of the Coliban Main Channel eastwards from its junction with the old Harcourt Channel.

'Passing Porter's Tunnel, half a mile further, brought me to the commencement of the Sandhurst section, which I will now begin to describe from its starting-point up to the Crusoe Gully Reservoir. In the first place, it will be as well to mention that from the starting-point of the Sandhurst channel, at the old eighteen mile peg up to No. 4 tunnel at thirty miles [48.2 km], with the single exception of No. 3 tunnel at twenty-five miles [40.2 km], this portion has been constructed within

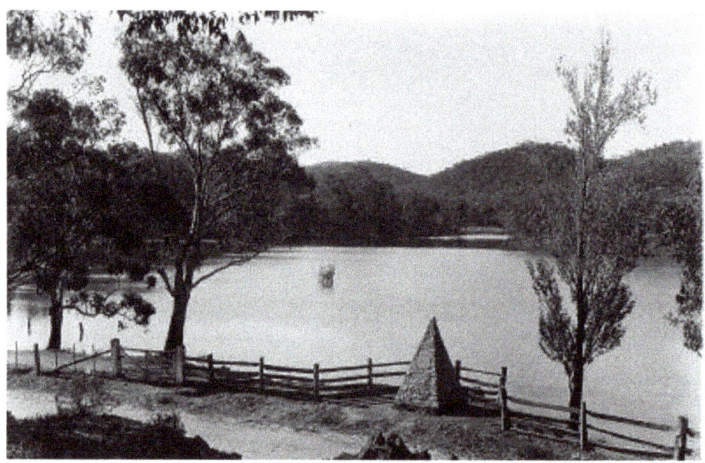

Expedition Pass Reservoir pre WWI. The monument in the foreground carries the inscription: 'On 20th September, 1836, Major Mitchell, after passing this ravine, named it Expedition Pass. Erected by public subscription 22nd April 1914.'

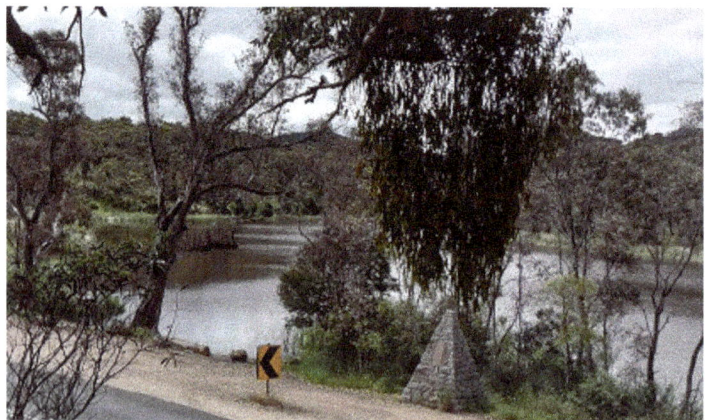

Present day view of the above location.

the last eighteen months, i.e. since June, 1876; and, therefore, I shall describe it as minutely as possible, and glance over the remainder to Crusoe Gully Reservoir, with only a short description of some of the principal features'.
Bendigo Advertiser, Tuesday 20 November 1877, p. 2.

While the short section from the channel's junction to the eastern side of the Calder Freeway isn't a difficult walk, the depth of water in the floodway under the freeway may be so great as to prevent easy access to the Sandhurst section of the main channel east of the freeway. It might be a safer bet to start the walk to Sutton Grange at Ellerys Lane (see map page 94).

> '... at the time of my visit a strong stream was flowing through the Castlemaine opening. From these gates the channel is lined with ashlar pitching and wings for a short distance, after which an open cutting of three chains in disintegrated granite brings it to a circular brick, and cement culvert, 3 feet 6 inches [1.1 m] in internal diameter, of 12 chains [241 m] in length, with

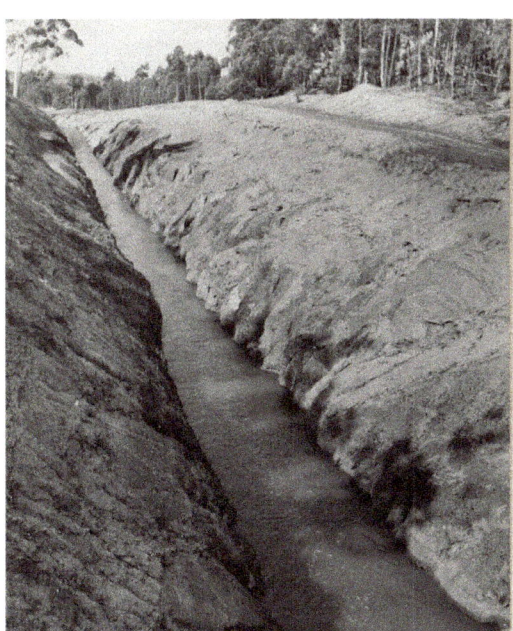 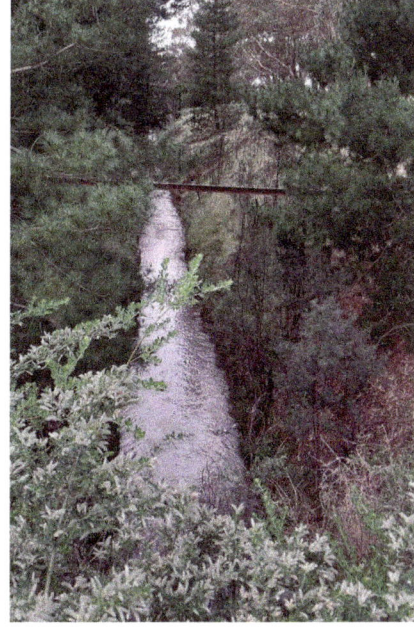

Site of old barrel culvert, Calder Highway, 1946, SR&WSC. Right: Present day view, Harmony Way.

strong, serviceable-looking, brick fronts and copings of granite. This culvert has a fall of 5 feet per mile, passing under the Melbourne road, and through a high spur. Its size appears very small in comparison with Porter's Tunnel, on the Castlemaine channel ... which struck me as being excessively large ...'
Bendigo Advertiser, Tuesday 20 November 1877, p. 2.

The 1870s barrel culvert mentioned above was demolished sometime before 1946, and the deep cutting, which is still visible today, was excavated. All that's left of the barrel culvert is the odd brick and a number of granite copings which can be seen inside the pine plantation close to Harmony Way.

After the deep cutting the channel waters flow again within a concrete race. After passing under a bridge the channel enters a culvert which takes it under the freeway.

For those who intend to follow the channel from the west side, the easiest path is to walk along Charles Lane, cross the bridge and bypass the gate. Nearby is a tunnel leading under the freeway. But be prepared to backtrack if the water level is high!

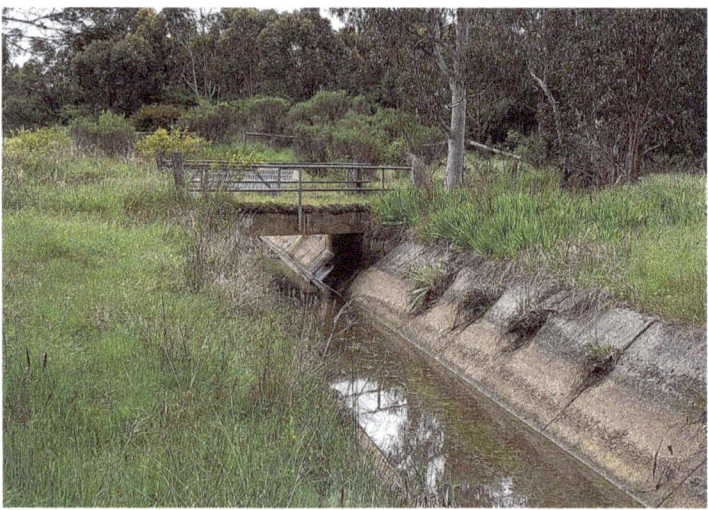

Bridge to floodway tunnel.

To one side of the tunnel there's a metal ledge with tree branches attached. This is designed to make it easier for wildlife to get through. If only the designers had included some stepping stones for us human animals.

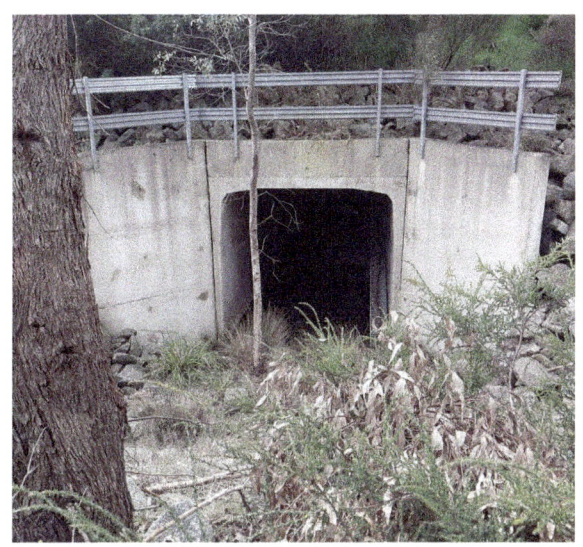

Floodway underpass.

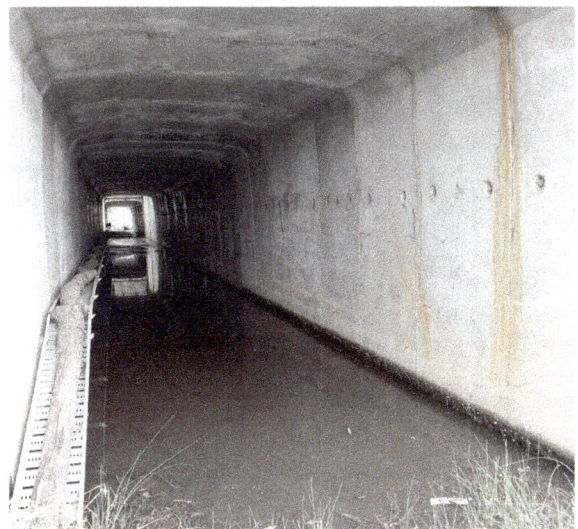

The underpass can be a bit damp at times!

Ellerys Road, Faraday to Faraday-Sutton Grange Road

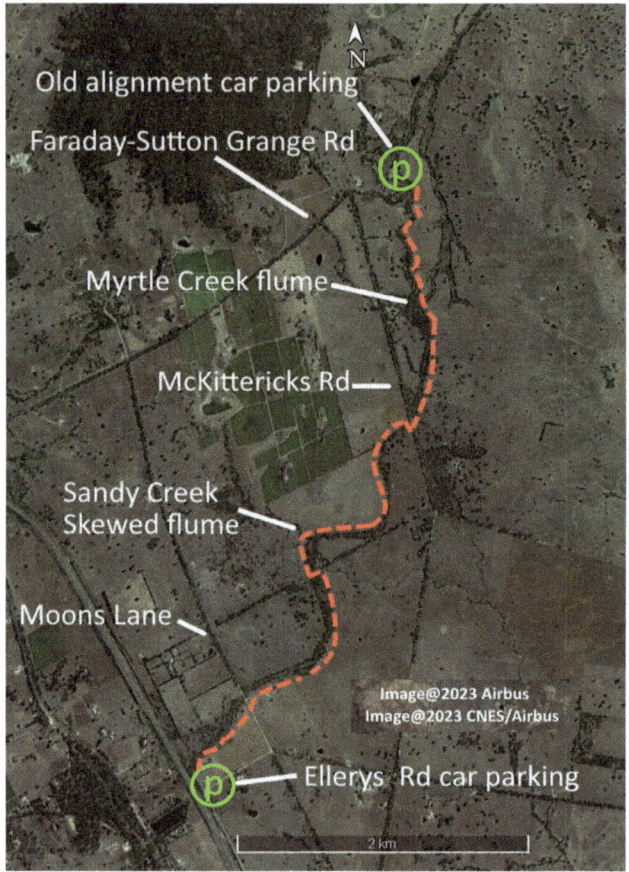

As the access track here is reasonably well maintained and easy to follow, this walk presents no great obstacles. But, again, this walk is best if a car shuttle can be arranged. One car should be parked just off to the side of Ellerys Road near the Calder Freeway, the other on an old alignment of the Faraday-Sutton Grange Road. This walk is about 6.5 km (double that if returning to Ellerys Lane).

The walk starts at Ellerys Lane near the Calder Freeway. There's a gate to negotiate, after which you should head north

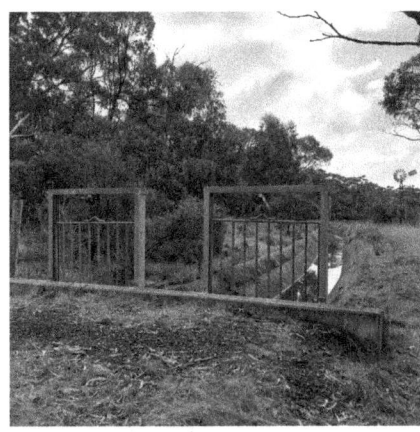

Culvert outlet, near Ellerys Road.

parallel to the freeway to reach the place where the channel emerges from a culvert. Turning east you soon reach Moons Lane. Here there are more gates to climb, or open and close (although most will be locked).

A bit further on, at an old road reserve, you will need to cross to the north side of the channel. About 1.5 km from Moons Lane you will arrive at Sandy Creek, notable for it being the site of a skew flume. It's quite a challenge to get to the other side of the channel to see the ruins of this flume. There is a sluice-gate (raised when the flow is stopped in the channel) which you can climb up and over, but the blackberries on the east side are gradually smothering the flume piers and abutments.

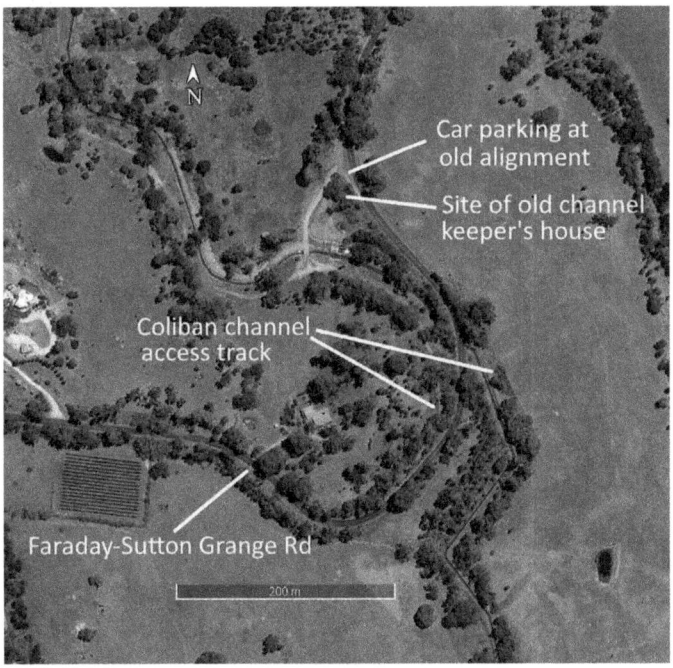

Detail of Faraday-Sutton Grange Road car parking.

'From the culvert before-named the water is carried a distance of a mile and a quarter in an open channel, at the end of which it enters a skew flume, built of timber, resting on masonry piers. This flume carries the water across Sandy Creek, a stream that flows into the Coliban River near Metcalfe. It runs at an elevation of seventeen feet [5.2 m] above the creek, and is 180 feet [54.9 m] long. The framework is constructed of red gum, and the trough which carries the water of red deal. In all cases the troughs of the flumes are kept constantly full of water by means of sliding boards inserted at the outlet end. This precaution is taken so as to prevent shrinkage.'
The Age, Thursday 3 January 1878, p. 3.

'The next work of any consequence in section 1 is the Sandy Creek flume at 19½ miles [31.4 km]. This structure is built on the skew, and is the only one of the kind along the channel. The framing is of red gum, apparently of very excellent character, resting on strong piers, of granite ashlar masonry,[31] built to a height of 18 inches above the ordinary water level of the creek and natural surface of the ground. The trough which carries the water is constructed of Oregon deal timber, the sides of 5 x 2 inch and bottom of 5 x 3 inch, tongued and grooved, and fitted with galvanised iron tongues, wrapped in green baize thoroughly soaked in tar, and the whole is firmly kept together by inside frames and wedges, which latter can be driven up or tightened, if required, on the timber shrinking. Each end is built into massive granite ashlar masonry abutments, with which a thoroughly watertight joint has been made. ...Its dimensions are 155 feet [47.2 m] long;[32] ... and it is designed to carry 2 feet in depth of water, with a fall of about 20 feet per mile.'
Bendigo Advertiser, Tuesday 20 November 1877, p. 3,

'... we turned from the confluence of the Sandhurst and Castlemaine races, along the course of the former until we came to the No. 1 or skew flume, as they call it. Here we found Mr. M. Lachlan, one of the officers in charge of the channel, up

---

31 Ashlar granite is masonry using blocks of stone that have been dressed to allow a close fit. Refer: Andrew p. 72.

32 Note the discrepancies between the two reporters in their measurement of the Sandy Creek flume.

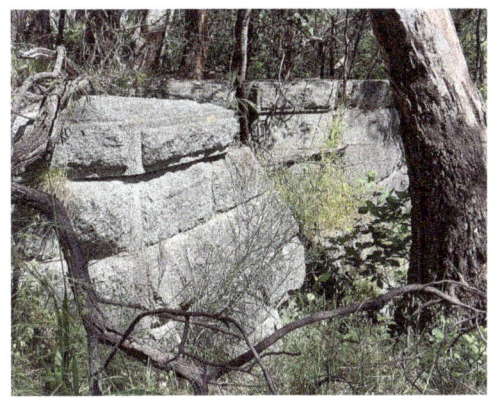

Sandy Creek flume abutments.

to his eyes, I was going to say, but a good deal over his ankles, in silt, which he was laboriously removing. There was a leak in the flume, which, during the time we stayed underneath it for the sake of the shade it afforded, was effectually stopped by himself and his assistant. When this was done we went with him to his abode.[33] Just here a really magnificent sight meets the view. We are at the head of Myrtle creek, and overlooking the fine and expansive valley known as Sutton Grange'.
Bendigo Advertiser, 26 November 1881 p. 1.

At McKittericks Road, turn right and cross over to the other side of the channel to resume your walk along the access track. Not far from here there is another demolished barrel culvert, like the one near Harmony Way.

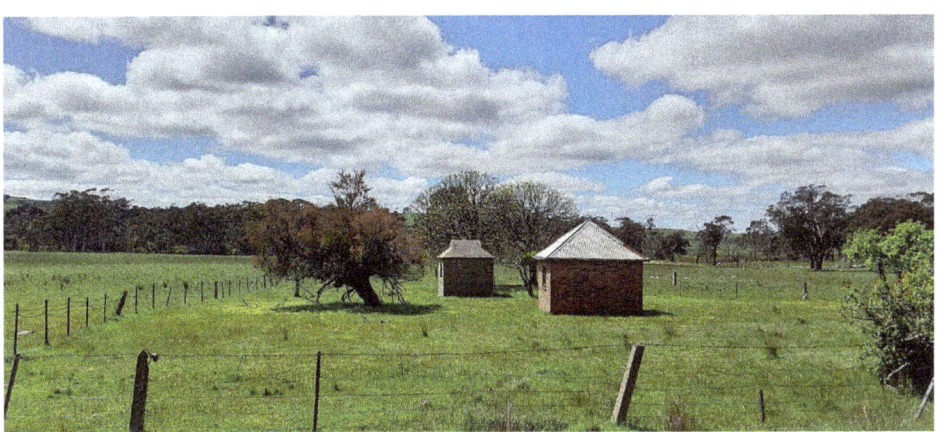

Looking east from Coliban Main Channel access track.

---

33 For the location of the Sutton Grange channel keeper's house, see page 102.

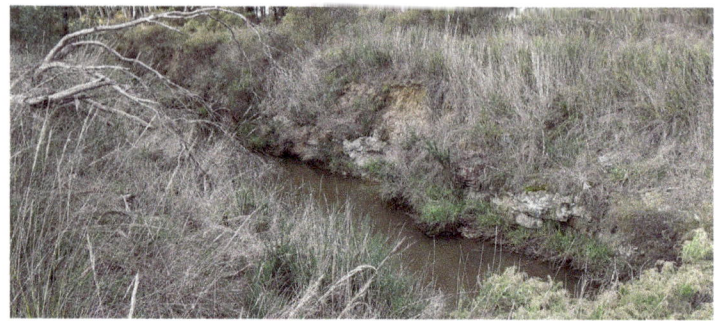

Site of demolished barrel culvert.

'Three-quarters of a mile [1.2 km] beyond this cutting, shortly before arriving at the Myrtle Creek flume, the channel passes through a high ridge (composed of very sandy material with a few bars of stiff clay and cemented sand intermixed) by means of a brick culvert. Some trial shafts put down before the works were commenced, showed that to form an open channel through this ridge would be very expensive, both as to first cost and subsequent maintenance, by reason of the very flat slopes that the material would require.

It was eventually decided by the engineer-in-chief to cut a trench and build a barrel culvert similar to that at the starting point, which was done. The carrying out of this work proved the wisdom of his plan, as considerable difficulty was experienced in keeping the trench open while the brick work was being executed. The length of this culvert is 13 chains [262 m], of circular form, 3½ feet in diameter, and with strong serviceable fronts like the other. Its average depth below the natural surface is about 15 feet, whilst the maximum is about 20 feet.'
Bendigo Advertiser, Tuesday 20 November 1877, p. 3.

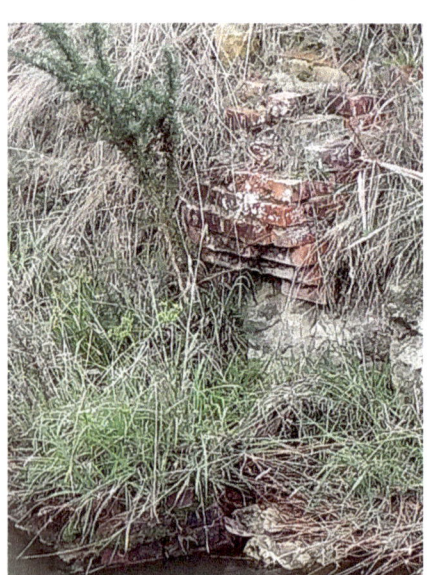

Close up of barrel culvert inlet ruins.

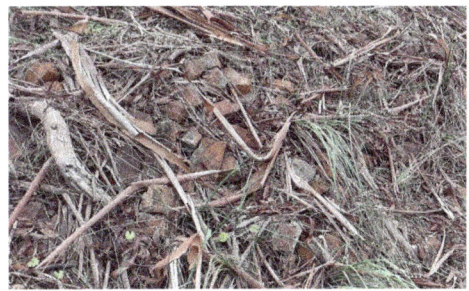
Bricks from the old barrel culvert at Myrtle Creek.

One of the features of this section of the channel is the picturesque nature of the old bypassed channel. It shows how important these wetlands and waterways are for aquatic vegetation and the reptiles and frogs that inhabit these backwaters.

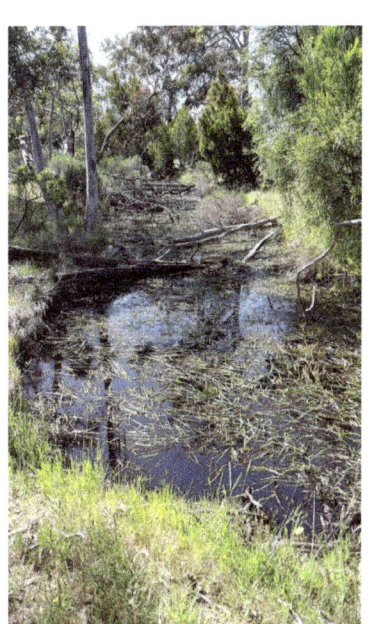
Bypassed channel near McKittericks Road.

'Proceeding on to Myrtle Creek, which is a little over 21 miles [33.8 km] on the channel, another timber flume similar to that last described spans the creek at a height of 34 feet from its bed. Its length is 400 feet [122 m], but there was one thing I observed for which there may have been good reasons, and that was that the timbers, instead of resting on masonry piers as at the other flume, were let into the ground without any protection from the action of the water. To my mind it seems a pity that masonry piers have not been used here, as the timber is sure to rot and require repairing in a short time, and as the material for them is handy this oversight is the more blameable...

I would here remark that during my inspection of the channel I was carefully on the lookout for the cause of the water being kept from running into Sandhurst, and could see no other point not complete, except the flume at Sandy Creek, before described. It appears to me, however, that an energetic contractor could easily finish this work sufficiently to allow of the water passing in 24 hours, as the work was evidently near its completion when I inspected it. From what I could learn on the spot, the Department has been pushing the contractor for the job for a long time to get it finished, but

without avail, and the people of Sandhurst have to thank him for keeping them out of the much-needed addition to the water supply. The Department has also been suffering loss by this contractor's culpable delay, as during the recent hot weather the flumes that are completed suffer from not being kept full of water.'
Bendigo Advertiser, Tuesday 20 November 1877, p. 3.

Very little of the Myrtle Creek flume has survived. The inlet abutments have collapsed into a gully and the outlet abutments are in ruins as well.

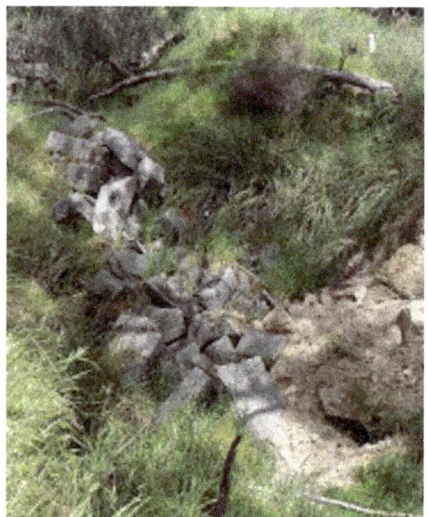 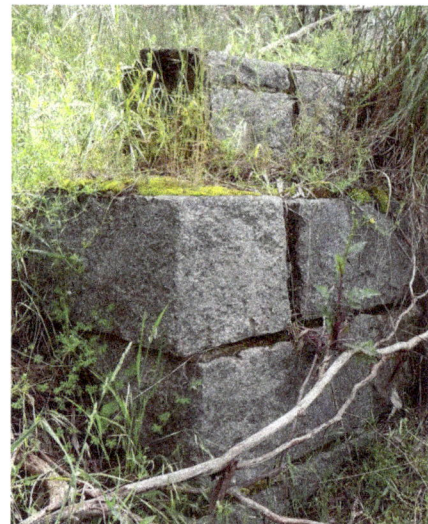

Ruins of flume inlet abutments. Right: outlet flume abutments.

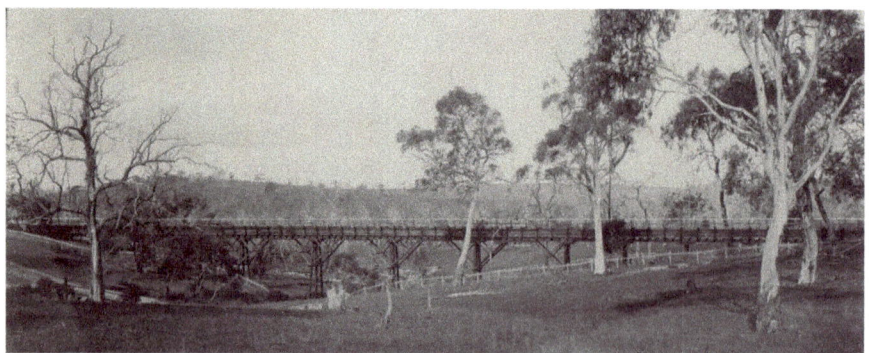

Myrtle Creek flume, looking east Photo: Kyneton Historical Society

One of the games I've enjoyed while walking the channel is to try to discover where a historic photo was taken, often with very few clues (the name of the exact location having long been lost). The photo below, showing how the channel was excavated, is a case in point. The State Library label leads one to think it's near the Malmsbury Reservoir. However, by looking at the photograph carefully we can narrow the options down until we find a place on the channel which matches it. In this case the trees have grown too much to obtain the same view, but I believe the photo was taken between Myrtle Creek and the Faraday-Sutton Grange Road.

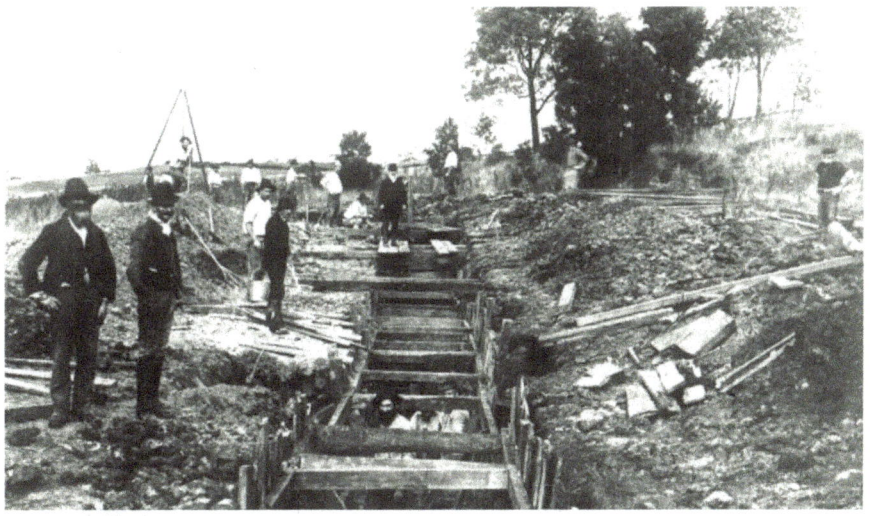

Excavating the Main Channel, 1870s. Below: Approximate site of the above location, Myrtle Creek vicinity.

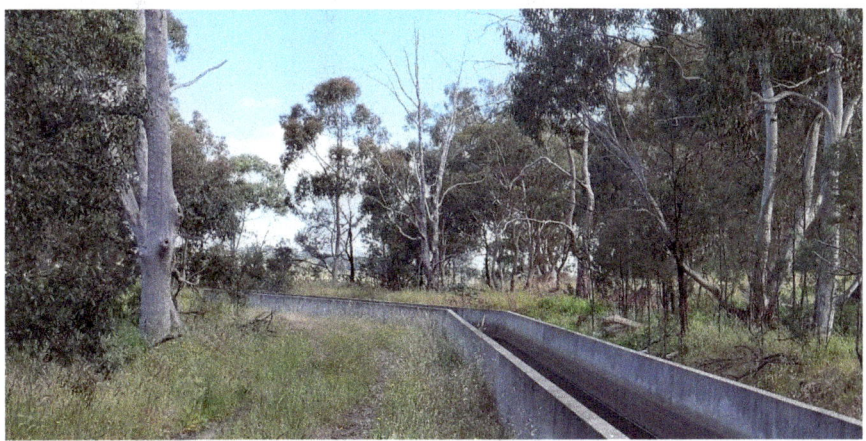

A few more twists and turns and the Faraday-Sutton Grange Road is just ahead. Once at the road you'll need to turn right and walk along the road shoulder, needless to say exercising a suitable degree of caution. If you've organised a car shuttle, your car should be straight ahead, in the old alignment of the road.

> 'At the Sutton Grange road the channel passes under it by means of a very fine circular brick culvert 3½ feet in diameter, and ornamented with granite copings, etc. The polluted water from the road is conveyed across the channel by a very lightly-constructed brick overshoot, with supporting arch underneath, and lined with cement. This is the only overshoot of the kind so far as I could see, and seems to answer the purpose remarkably well, the others being principally of red gum, and occasionally earthenware pipes.
>
> This takes us into section 2, where, close to the channel, a keeper's three-roomed cottage has been built, which at present answers the purpose of the engineer's office on the works.'
> *Bendigo Advertiser, Tuesday 20 November 1877, p. 3.*

Fronting this short bypassed section of the Faraday-Sutton Grange Road very little of this house remains, although a very wild and weed infested garden gives a clue as to where the house was

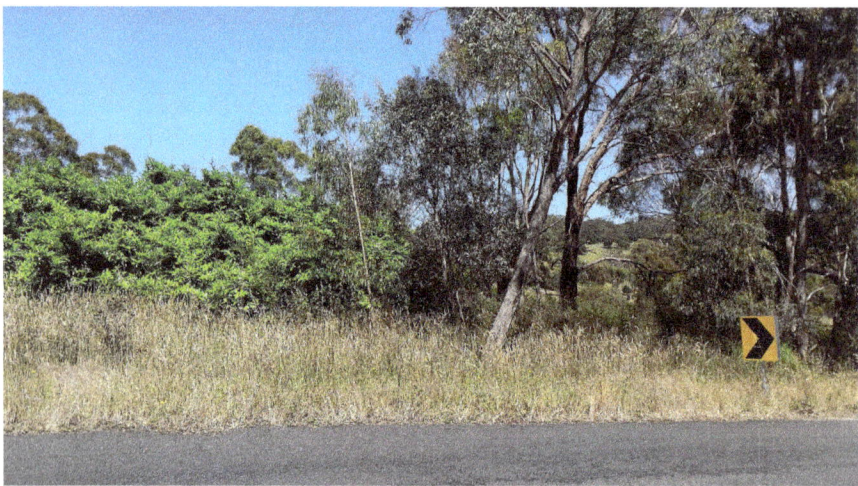

Site of the Sutton Grange channel keeper's (water bailiff) house and the original site office of Coliban Channel works.

situated. Apparently the house was removed to Harcourt in the late '80s or early '90s.[34] One small memento remains, probably a chicken coop.

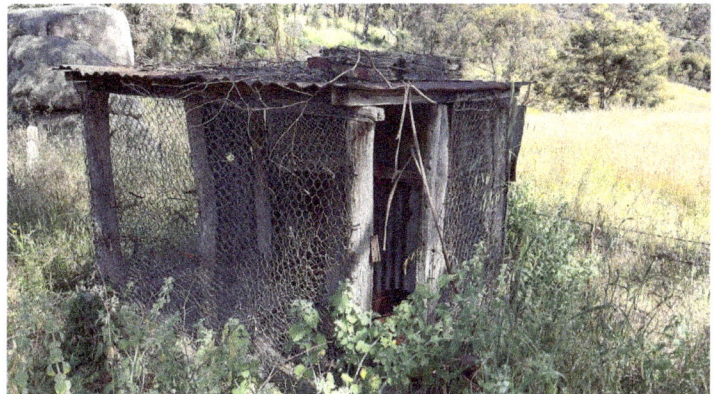

Chicken coop or rabbit hutch? Old channel keeper's house (later a water bailiff) Sutton Grange.

'I have said that the scenery at the head of Myrtle Creek is very fine and well worth the journey. By a steep descent from the place of its source, it falls into a fine wide fertile valley, which opens out beyond the limit of one's view, until it is lost in the plains skirting the western bank of the Coliban. Looking in that direction, the eye roams over a very interesting park-like country, studded with pretty farmsteads, whilst the little postal village known as Myrtle Creek lies hidden beneath the surrounding hills, and seven miles further on is that of Sutton Grange. Turning to the ranges overlooking the vale one discovers much that is interesting, even romantic, and highly picturesque.

    The mountain side is full of what I suppose Professor Denton[35] would call "wrinkles," and indeed the old hill is very deeply furrowed with them. ... Here we see gum trees of giant

---

34 Noel Davis, personal communication via Facebook History Group.
35 In the 1870s, Professor William Denton earned a reputation as one of Australia's leading public educators. In October 1881, he delivered a series of well-attended lectures on geology in Bendigo. Sadly, within just two years he was dead from a tropical illness caught on an expedition to New Guinea. *Australian Town and Country Journal*, 20 October 1883, p. 25.

height and proportions dwarfed in the great granitic clefts by their bold and lofty surroundings. These glens or gorges are full of springs; consequently the vegetation in their bottoms is rank, thick, and tangled; but always pretty, sometimes beautiful, and ever green.

I confess I could spend a week with much pleasure on the eastern slopes of Mount Alexander, wandering amongst the great precipitous rocks of granite, from a single one of which might be obtained, the material for building a city of mighty dimensions; gazing on the strange sights, the pleasing, grand, and ever changing views presenting themselves at every turn; and pondering on the terrible convulsions which mother earth in this part must have undergone in a long bye gone age.'
Bendigo Advertiser, Saturday 3 December 1881, p. 1.

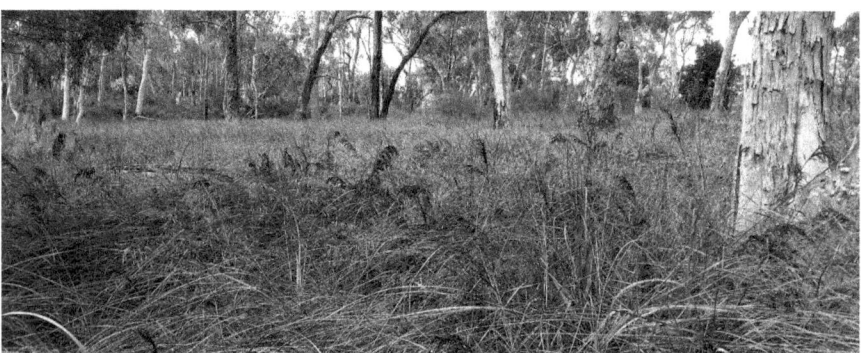

Myrtle Creek flume environs, present day view.

Faraday-Sutton Grange Road to Harcourt-Sutton Grange Road

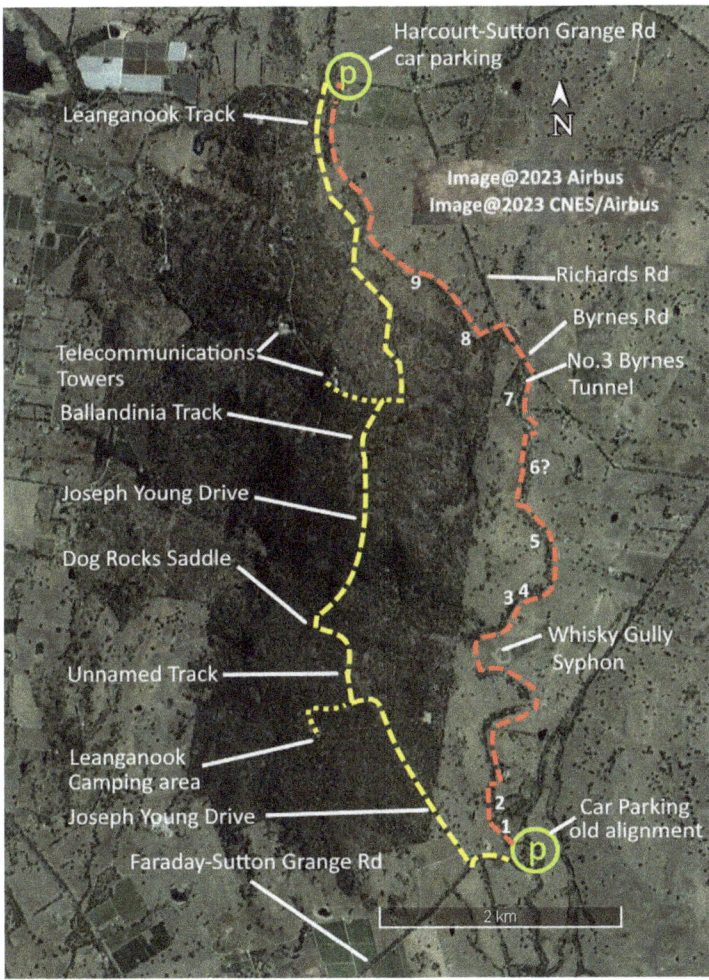

This is probably the most scenic of the walks described in this book (one-way it's about 9 km). Nineteenth century writers who visited the east side of Mount Alexander were struck both by the beauty of the region and the ambitious engineering structures that were erected here to convey the Coliban water across the numerous gullies and ravines. The numbers on the map indicate the locations of timber flumes detailed in the track notes.

The walk is best done by utilising a car shuttle, one car parked at the previously described old alignment of the Faraday-Sutton Grange Road and the other in the large if highly eroded car park next to the channel at the Harcourt-Sutton Grange Road. A return walk of about 20 km can be made by coming back through the Mount Alexander Regional Park, but it would require an early start as well as a dangerous final stretch along the shoulder of the Faraday-Sutton Grange Road. Walkers could make a two day walk of it by camping overnight at the Leanganook Camping Area off Joseph Young Drive (see map previous page). As the walk back through the Regional Park is complicated, with tracks often poorly marked and maintained, it is vital that a more detailed map be used for navigation purposes. A printable map of the Mount Alexander Regional Park can be downloaded from Jase Haysom's excellent Cartography Community Mapping website: ccmaps.au

Step through the wire fence next to the gate at the car parking area at the old alignment of the Faraday-Sutton Grange Road and follow the channel access track northwards. The track has recently been metalled and widened to accommodate machinery that was called in to repair a section of concrete channelling.

> '... the second section, of three miles [4.8 km] in length, is of a very rugged character, and my pen can but faintly portray the many engineering difficulties that had to be overcome in winding the channel around the eastern slope of Mount Alexander, here between rocks and boulders, there over steep spurs, and again across deep valleys.

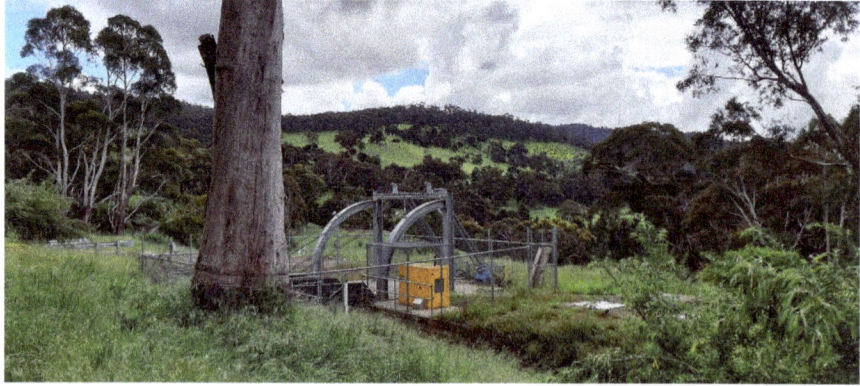

Trash grate (and ringbarked tree), Sutton Grange (Mount Alexander is in distance).

Of the three miles embraced by this section I believe there is about half a mile of the massive granite walling before referred to, about one-third of a mile of an inverted syphon, nearly a third of a mile [805 m] of flumes, about a quarter of a mile [402 m] of cutting through solid granite rock, from 2 to 6 feet deep, and about a mile and three-quarters [2.8 km] of ordinary cutting through disintegrated granite, moderately heavy granite rock, and huge boulders. These walls are, on an average, about 2 feet thick, of rock-faced granite-squared masonry. They appear about three feet above the bottom of the channel generally, and most of them are stepped into the solid rock upon which they are built. They present a very good appearance, and are said to be cheaper than excavating the channel out of the solid rock.'

'The flumes in this section are seven in number.[36] The first rests entirely on granite abutments and piers, the troughs of which, together with those of the remaining six, are of a similar character to those already described as passing over Sandy and Myrtle creeks.'

Bendigo Advertiser, Tuesday 20 November 1877, p. 3.

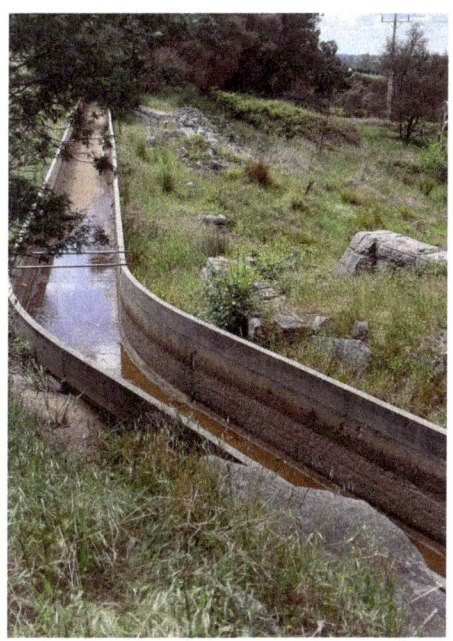

Flume 1: flume abutments, seen here to the right of the current channel.

'It may here be mentioned that it was at one time confidently asserted that the granite formation on the Mount Alexander slopes would never hold water, but experience has shown that it does, subject to as little percolation as any other kind of formation along the line of the aqueduct. Indeed, I may state that it was only here and there, at long distances apart, that I observed slight weepings, caused no doubt by the water finding

---

36 These are numbered 1 to 7 on the map (page 105) and in the text and photos.

its way through some vein in the rock. In the course of time the sediment from the water will fill up those crevices, and the drain will become watertight'
The Age, Thursday 3 January 1878, p. 3.

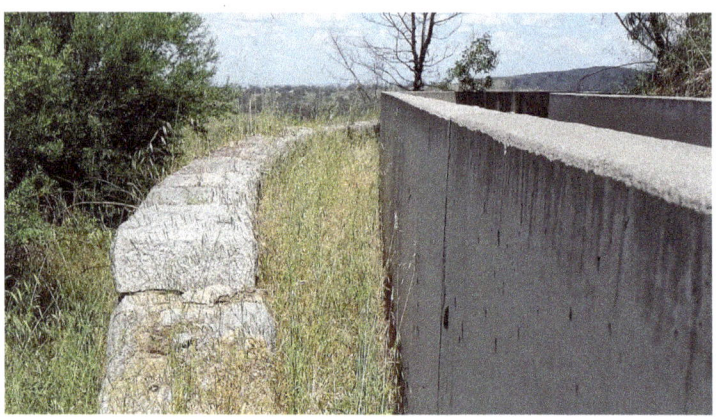
Later concrete channel constructed alongside earlier ashlar granite wall.

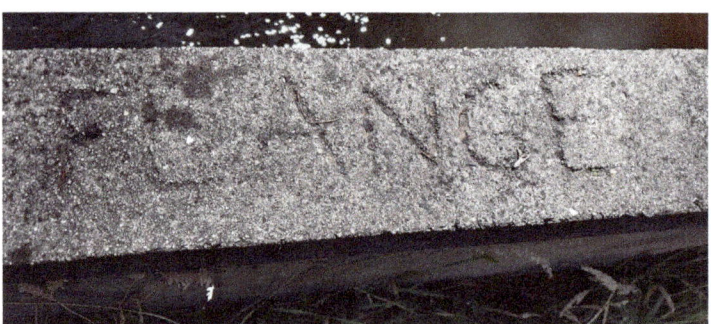
Who was Flange?

Along the channel in this section a group of men inscribed their names into the top of a freshly cemented channel wall. Max, Ivor, Bourkey and the enigmatic Flange!

> 'The second flume rests on masonry and timber piers, all of which are set into the natural rock. One end of this flume passes between two huge boulders, the natural space between which had been increased to admit it.'
> *Bendigo Advertiser, Tuesday 20 November 1877, p. 3.*

'There is a fall of 290 feet [88.4 m] from the eighteen mile peg at Expedition Pass to Pall Mall, Sandhurst, and along the course there are sixteen flumes, the shortest of which is ninety-three feet [28.3 m], and the longest 650 feet [198 m]. They vary in height from ten to forty feet [12.2 m] above the level of the ground. In the short space of three miles on the Mount Alexander slopes there are about 1700 feet [518 m] of fluming. The country through which the channel passes is parklike, hilly

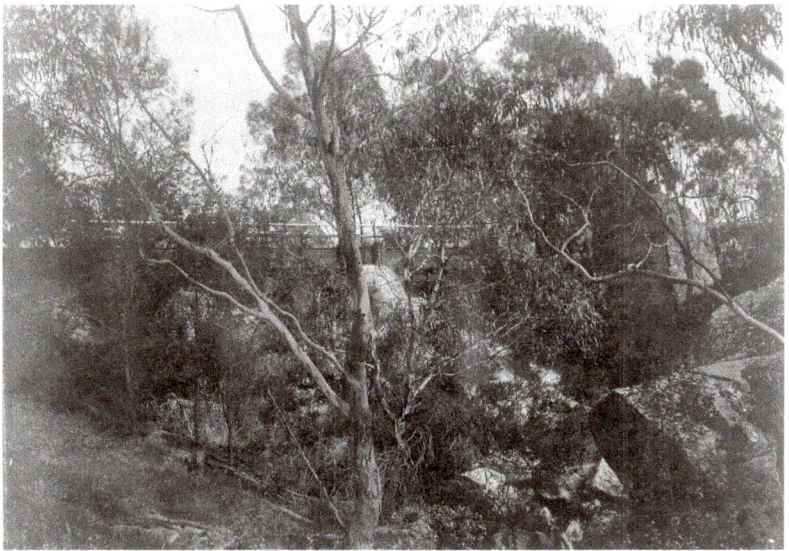

Flume 2: an undated photograph, probably ca. 1900.

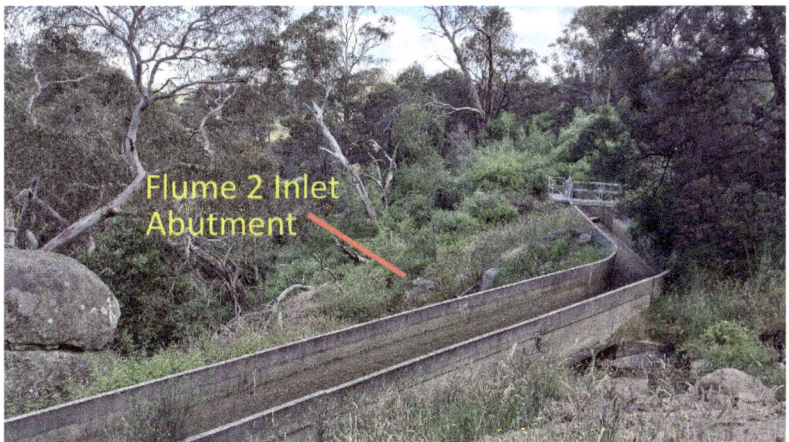

Location of Flume 2.

and picturesque. Much of it is well adapted for potato culture, and nearly all of it, if under cultivation, requires irrigation.'
The Age, Thursday 3 January 1878, p. 3.

Cattle appear to freely roam the Coliban reserve but seem willing to return to their pastures when disturbed. In many places the boundary fences have collapsed and have yet to be repaired. Walkers should exercise care and refrain from scaring the cattle to the point of panic.

It might be thought that there should have been two parallel 1870s ashlar granite walls rather than just one as is the case here. The argument was that as water is unlikely to flow uphill, the wall was there simply to hold the flowing water on its course. In some cases the concrete channel has been erected on the uphill side of the old wall. However, at other locations, such as here, the old wall is above the newer channel.

Once, the channel waters would have flown to the right of this wall with only the ground slope to confine the water.

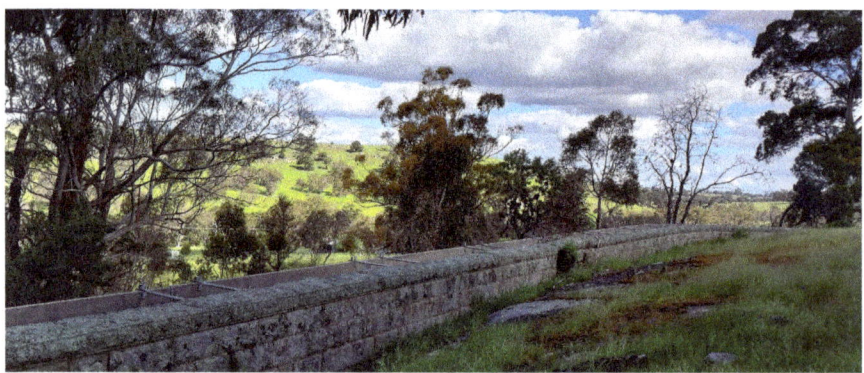

Granite wall built in 1876.

'A cast-iron inverted syphon,[37] over a third of a mile [536 m] in length, will carry the water across a deep ravine (near the "Silk Farm")[38] which is one of the tributaries of Myrtle Creek. The

---

37 This syphon was doubled in 1905. *The Bendigo Independent*, Monday 2 October 1905, p. 3.

38 The Victorian Ladies Sericulture Company tried to develop a silkworm industry on Mount Alexander between 1874 and 1878, but the site proved unsatisfactory. The ruins of the granite buildings still remain. *The Argus*, Saturday 23 February 1878, p. 8.

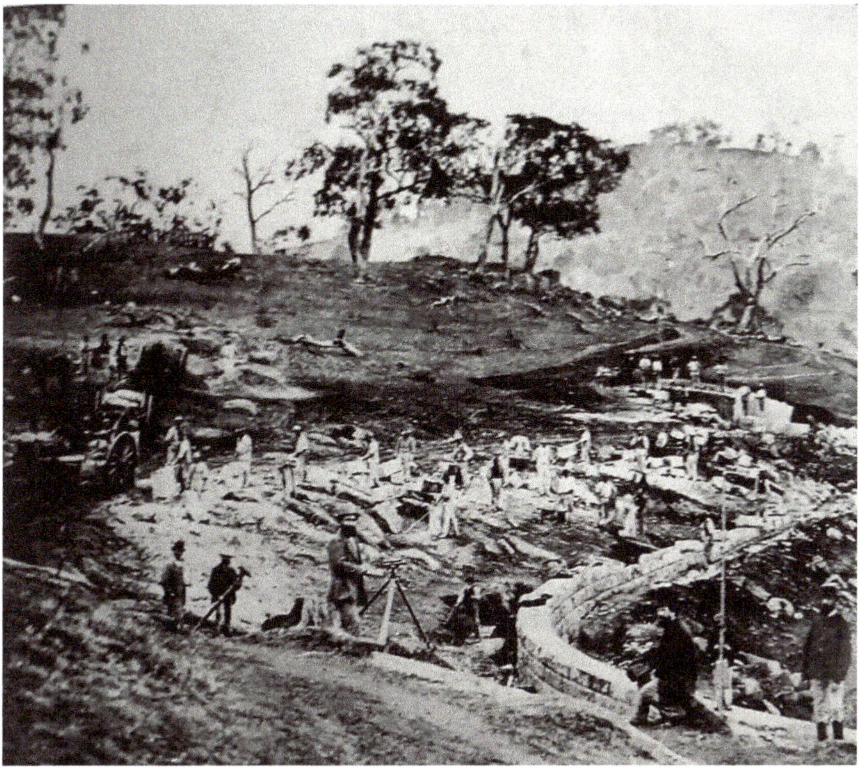

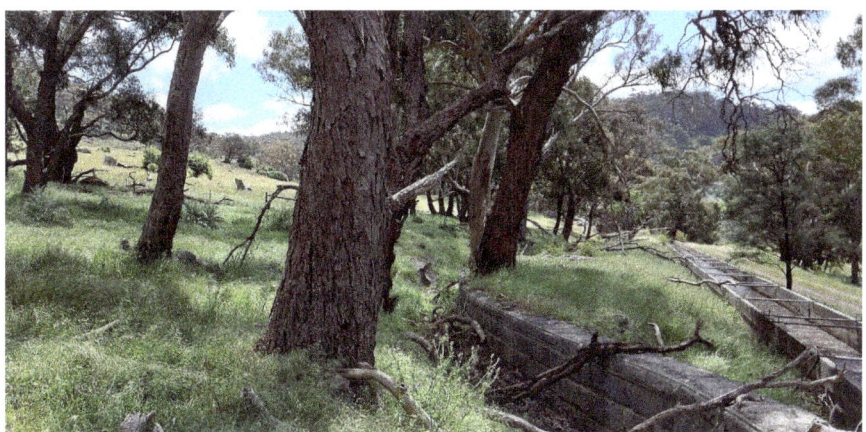

Channel near Whisky Gully (a tributary of Myrtle Creek) syphon, 1876.

Present day view.

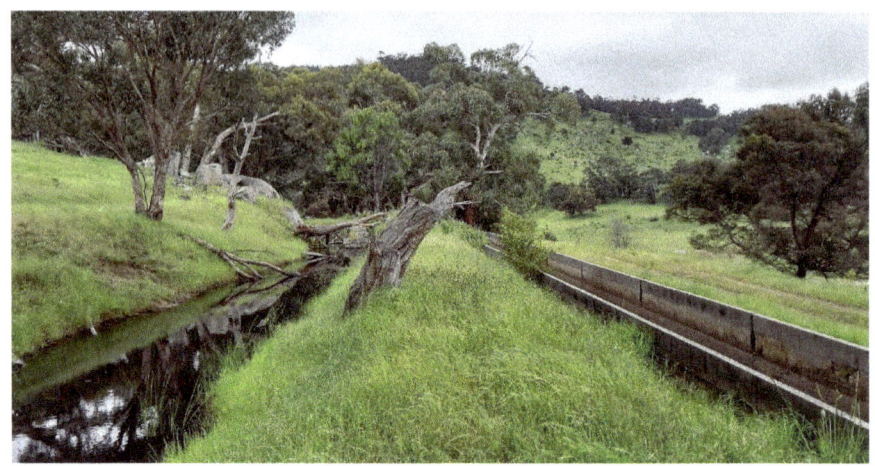
The old channel on the left, the later channel on the right.

> inverted syphon is 27 inches in internal diameter, and is laid about 2 feet under the surface, down the slope of the gully, across the creek (which is a tributary of Myrtle Creek), and up the opposite slope. ... At the entrance end the inlet works consist of very fine granite ashlar masonry, forming a circular tank, with wing walls fitted with screens, and the opening into the pipe is bell-mouthed. At the outlet end the masonry is of a similar character, being simply a cross-wall, with ramped wings. The whole of this portion of the work appears to have been executed with great care.'
> *Bendigo Advertiser, Tuesday 20 November 1877, p. 3,*

And so we come to the second great syphon installed in the Coliban Water Scheme. Whisky Gully is one of the deepest gullies encountered on the eastern side of Mount Alexander. The first solution was to run a cast iron pipe underground across the width of this wide gully (perhaps running under the large dam here). Later it was replaced by a much larger concrete syphon built above and across Whisky Gully closer to the head of the gully. Still later, an aqueduct was built on top of an embankment even closer to the head of the gully.

In the photo on the next page, you might be able to see a red excavator. This was called in to help repair a section of the channel which had collapsed during the heavy rain events of October 2022.

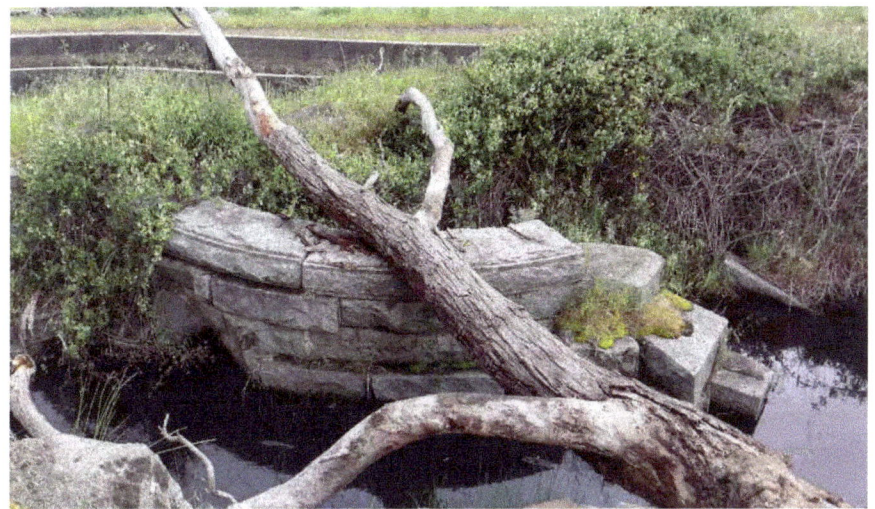
Inverted syphon inlet (Whisky Gully). Pity about that tree!

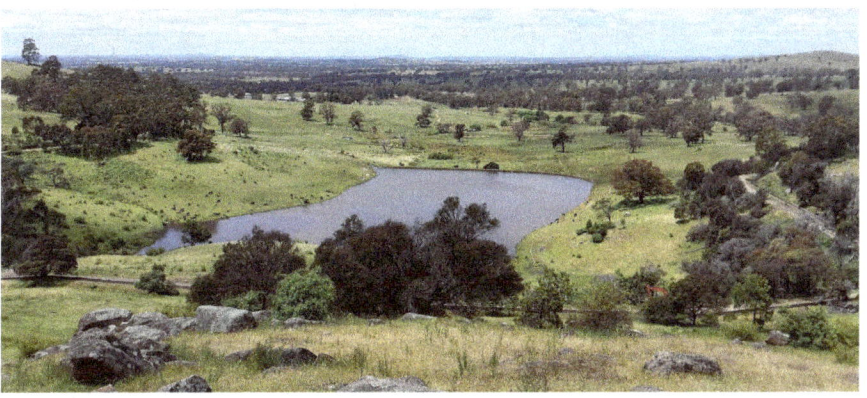
The view looking across Whisky Gully. The 1870s syphon is probably now buried beneath the waters of the dam in the middle distance.

There is a choice for walkers at Whisky Gully. You can continue to follow the access track as it descends and rises to the other side of the gully. Or you can follow the channel itself. It will mean walking along the edge of the aqueduct above the Whisky Gully gorge, but it provides excellent views of the concrete syphon, built in 1919 after it was decided to supersede the old cast iron syphon. After crossing the aqueduct, you can see a rather nondescript shaft leading down to the syphon pipe outlet.

After the access track is rejoined it isn't far until the remains of a double or skew flume is reached (Flumes 3 and 4).

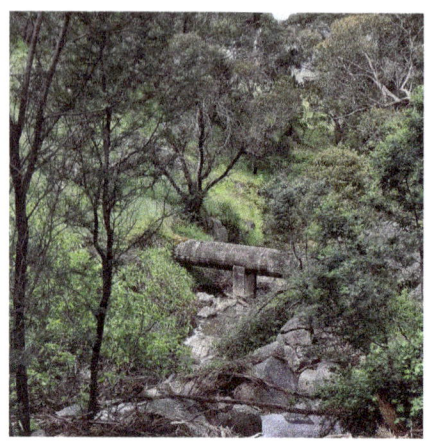 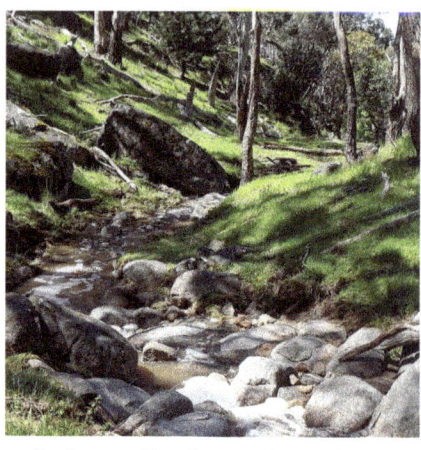

Second syphon (1919) Whisky Gully. *Whisky Gully above channel.*

'The third, fifth, and seventh flumes, which have the ordinary kind of masonry abutments and timber piers, resting on masonry foundations, span deep ravines, and the fourth and sixth are placed along steep sidling ground, along which one can hardly walk.'
Bendigo Advertiser, 20 November 1877, p. 3.

'The channel, after leaving the syphon mouth, is composed almost continuously for about a quarter of a mile [402 m] of an earthwork embankment, when it enters another skew flume. The first portion of this flume crosses a rugged valley at a considerable elevation, The remaining part of the aqueduct traverses for over a mile steep sideling ground supported on the lower side by a granite wall'
The Age, 3 January 1878, p. 3.

Along this section of the channel there are a number of gates to negotiate. However at one or two, a handy notched step has been placed to make it easier to climb over. Farm access tracks will also be encountered allowing cattle to cross between paddocks above and below the channel.

Further along, below the track, you will see the granite piers of another flume. I spent some time looking for the location of the 6th flume. The photo on page 117 shows the remains of it – a single granite abutment.

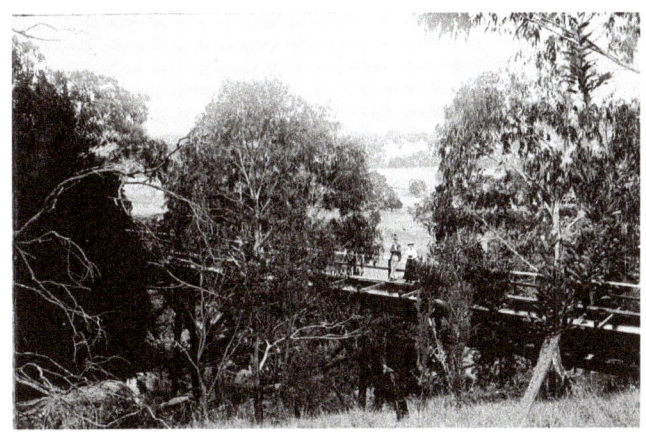

Flume 3: 1894 (looking east). Photographer M. Law.

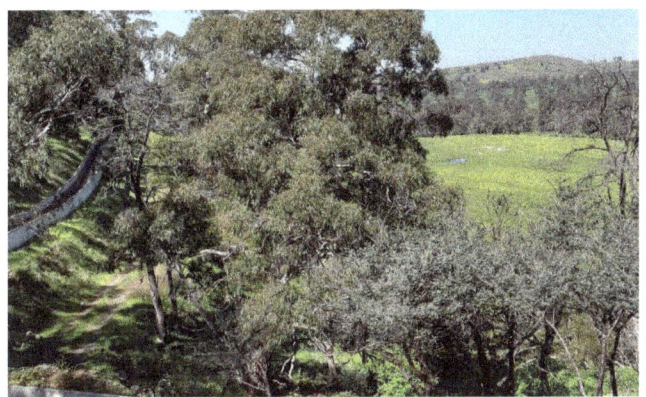

Location of Flume 3, looking east.

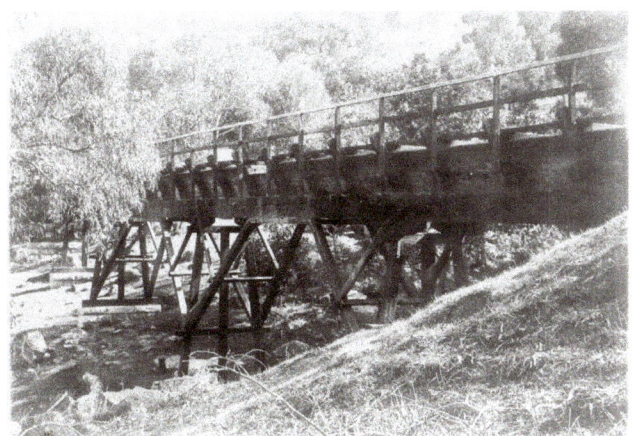

Flume 3: looking south-west.

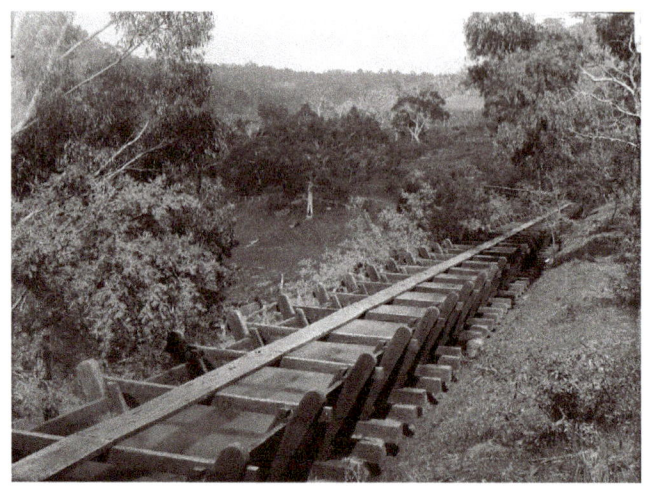

Flume 4: looking south 1900 (flume 3 in the distance).

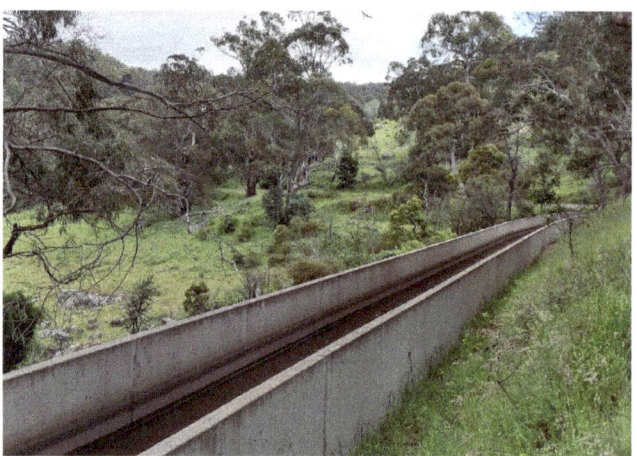

Present day view of the above location.

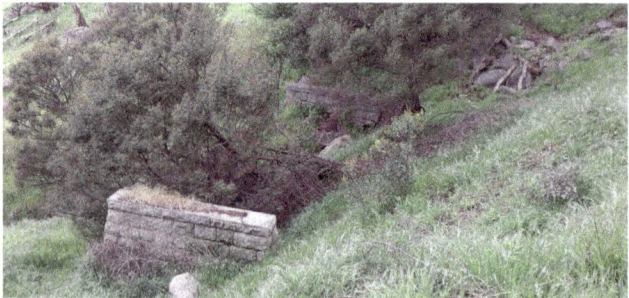

Flume 5: Granite piers.

Probably the most dramatic feature along the east side of Mount Alexander was flume 7. The engineering difficulties in constructing this flume are evident in the old photo on the following page.

The Byrnes family has long farmed just below this gully. They gave their name to a road, a tunnel and a quarry near here. One early photo gives the name of the flume as Byron's Flume. My theory is that it's a mishearing of Byrnes. Nowadays, the creek that flows, sometimes with extraordinary force through this gully, is called Byrnes Creek.

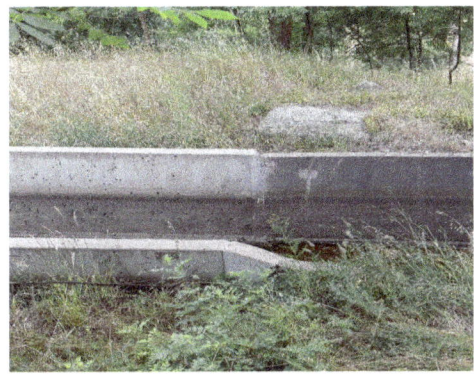

Site of Flume 6?

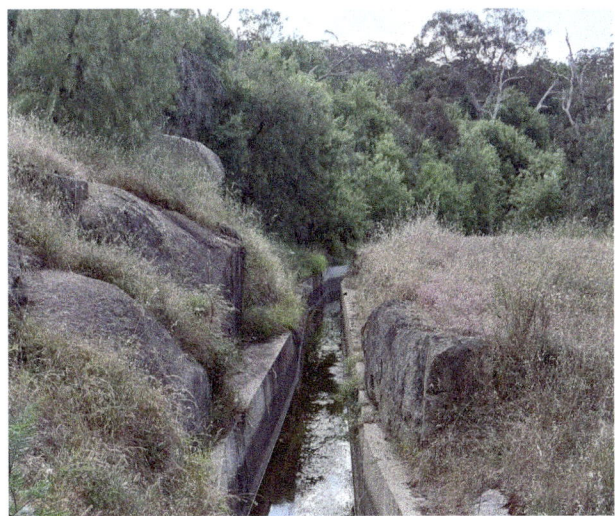

Channel leading up to Byrnes Creek.

'The last flume just before entering No. 3 tunnel, crosses a very picturesque valley studded with huge granite boulders. At this point the natural slope of the hillsides being about three or four to one great difficulty was experienced in getting materials necessary for the works along the ground to the required sites. In addition to this difficulty, advantage had to be taken of clear places along which to wind the channel between huge boulders, to have removed, which would have cost enormous sums of money. The skill displayed by Mr. Henderson in engineering the channel through this difficult country can hardly be too warmly praised.'
The Age, Thursday 3 January 1878, p. 3,

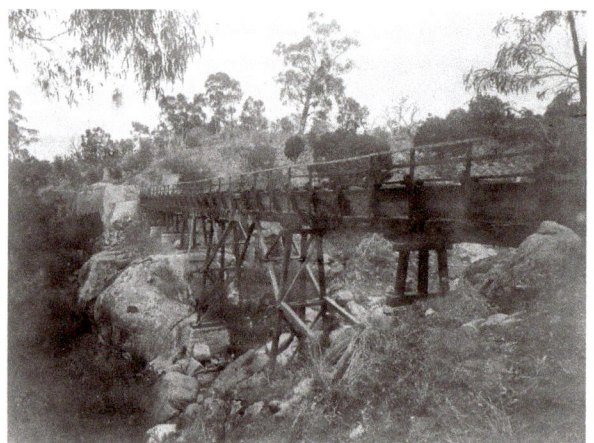

Flume 7: Byron's Flume (Byrnes Creek gully).

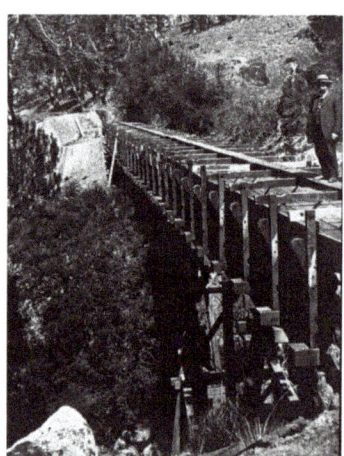

A later view of Byron's Flume ca. 1920.

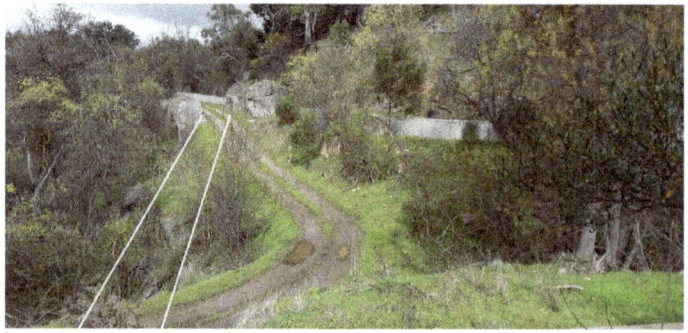

Site of Flume 7 today (with alignment of the original flume marked).

Within three hundred metres, the mouth of No. 3 (Byrnes) Tunnel is reached.

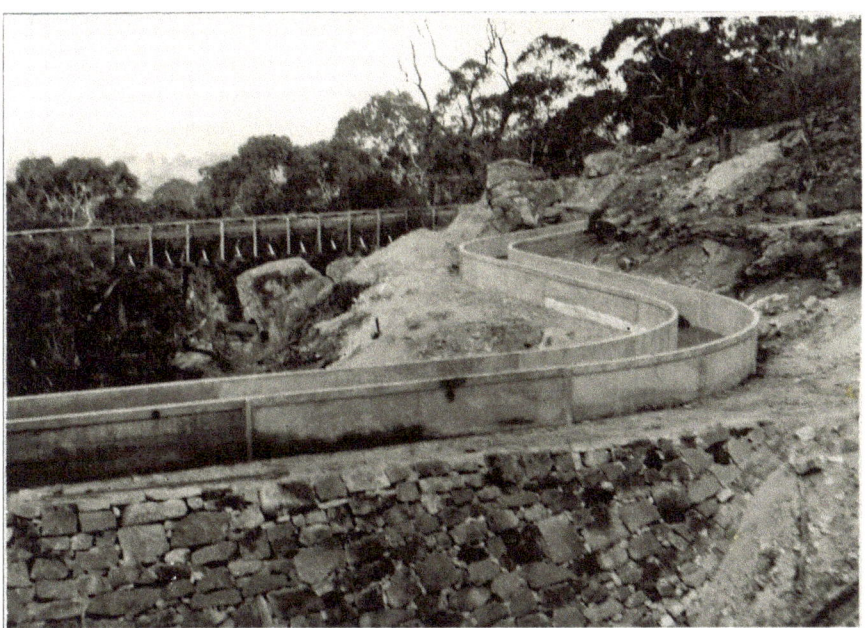

Construction of new aqueduct with old decommissioned flume behind. Photo courtesy of Bendigo Historical Society. Below: Present day view.

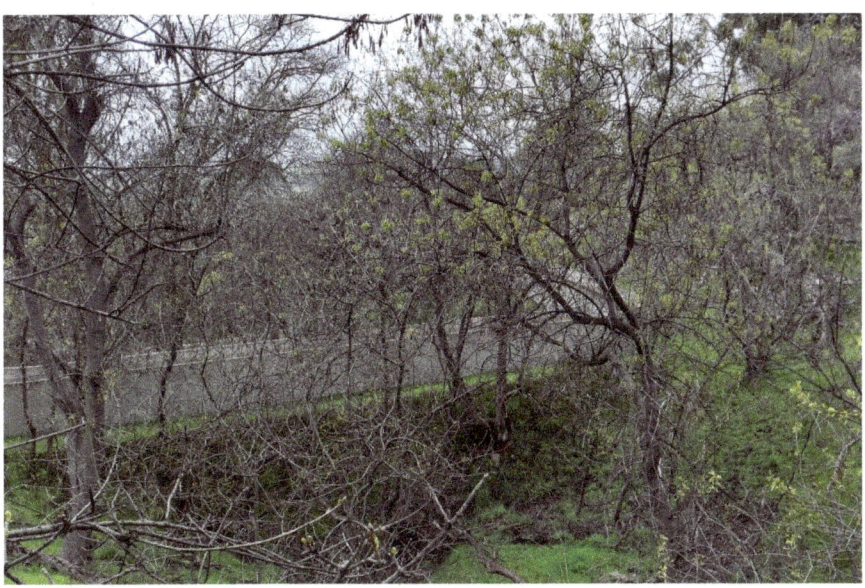

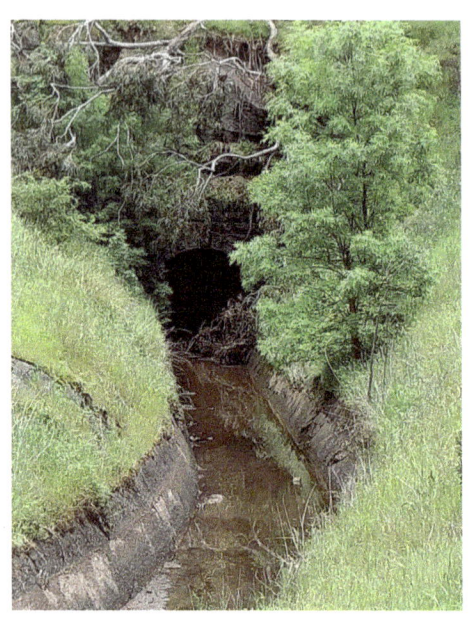
No. 3 (Byrnes) Tunnel entrance.

'We have now arrived at No. 3 tunnel,[39] which is an old work, of similar size to Porter's Tunnel, being 9 feet in diameter, at an elevation of 1,319 feet above the sea level, the summit of the hill through which it passes being 1,393 feet above sea level, and one can hardly see the utility of making it so large and spending such immense sums of money on a work that would have answered the purpose quite as well had it been made only half the size.

Indeed, from the size of the culverts already described it would appear that 3½ feet would have been ample, if the driving of such a sized tunnel would have been practicable. The length of this tunnel is about the eighth of a mile, and it has been driven mostly through granite. Some slight repairs and additions to the lining were going on when I was there, which was necessitated by a vein of soft material making across it.'
Bendigo Advertiser, Tuesday 20 November 1877, p. 3,

Once at Byrnes Road, turn left, climb up the hill and the road becomes Richards Road. Enter the gate about 500 metres on the left.

'After passing No. 3 tunnel the watercourse enters what is known as Wellington Flat. This locality consists of fine undulating, well-grassed country still on a granite formation. The land belongs to Mr. Richard Towers and Mr. J. Young, and, like other lands along the route, this area is well suited for irrigation, if it were used for crops requiring water. This flat, however, is intersected by one or two moderately deep and

---

39 Noel Davis says that there is a dip inside the tunnel where water collects when the flow is stopped. In the past, when this happened, fish trapped in this pool were collected by locals (personal communication).

rugged ravines, across which the water is carried by means of flumes. The channel for some further distance is carried along in [an] open ditch cut in moderately easy soil, and the gullies that have to be crossed present no engineering difficulties. It will be observed that in this locality several drops have been inserted, and on inquiry I found that the reason for so doing was that the sandy nature of the soil rendered them necessary in order to reduce the scour, by lessening the fall that obtains elsewhere. If the fall had not been reduced, the scour that prevails in sections that traverse harder formations would have been so strong that the sandy material of which the ground is composed would have been washed away. The width of the channel has been increased, as in other similar cases, so as to compensate for the slower rate at which the water travels.'
The Age, Thursday 3 January 1878, p. 3,

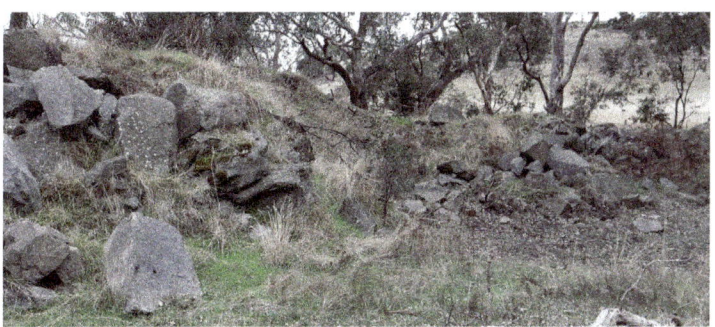

Byrnes Quarry.

Just inside the gate on the left is Byrnes Quarry, an old granite quarry. This was the source of some of the granite used along this part of the channel. Apparently, this area, Wellington Flat, was the site of a camp for the work crews whose task it was to begin the process of concreting the old earthen channels during the 1930s. This work was funded by the Government to provide work for unemployed men, the Great Depression having lingered for a long time in Australia.

> 'In a report to be submitted to the State Government shortly, the Public Works Committee will recommend the expenditure of £200,000 on the Coliban water system. Of this sum the

committee will recommend that £100,000 be spent in Bendigo on reticulation and remodelling; £50,000 in Castlemaine, and £50,000 on the lining of the main channels. The Coliban system supplies water to Bendigo, Castlemaine and other districts, but with the present earthen channels it is stated that one-third of the water is being lost in transit by seepage. The relining with concrete of the channels will save this water. Castlemaine, which will be sewered shortly, will be given a better water supply, and other districts will also benefit. Hundreds of men will be employed on the work.'
Weekly Times, Saturday 25 April 1936, p. 30.

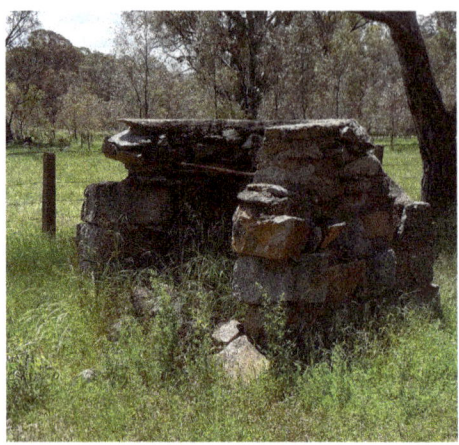
Fireplace, Wellington Flat.

Apparently, dances were held here for the susso workers[40] and locals during the 1930s.[41] A fireplace has survived, not far past the gate, perhaps from that time. It might make a good informal camping site for those not wishing to head up to the Leanganook Camping Area.

In about 200 metres there are the ruins of one of the grandest flumes of the entire Coliban Main Channel. This gully is a tributary of Axe Creek.

> 'The works on this section comprise open cuttings through rock, boulders and disintegrated granite, three flumes, bridges, waste weirs, and other works, the design of which, together with the open channel, is very similar to that described in section 1, and need not be repeated, as no engineering work of any note occurs in its course.'
> *The Bendigo Advertiser 20 November 1877 p. 2.*

---

40 Unemployed men working for sustenance.
41 Noel Davis, personal communication via Facebook History Group, August 18 2023.

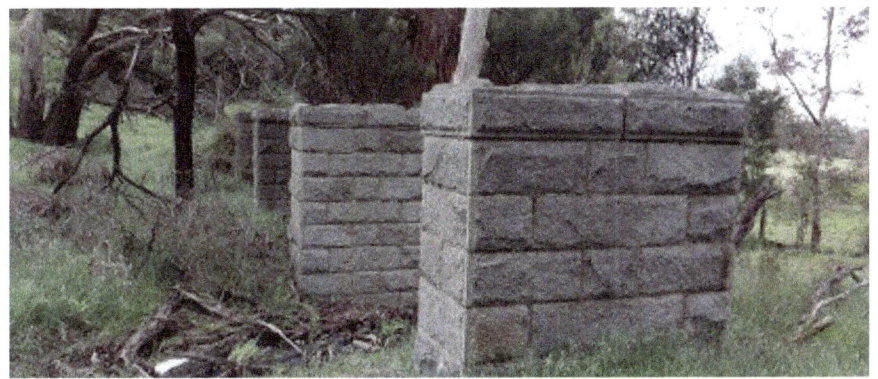

Flume piers: North of Richards Road, Axe Creek tributary. Below: Another view.

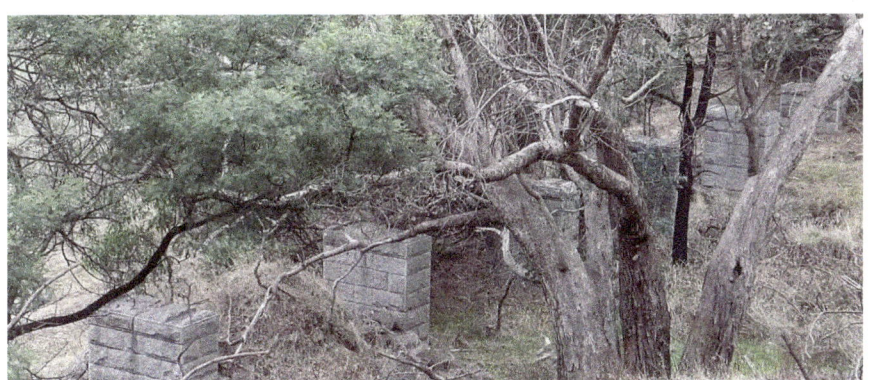

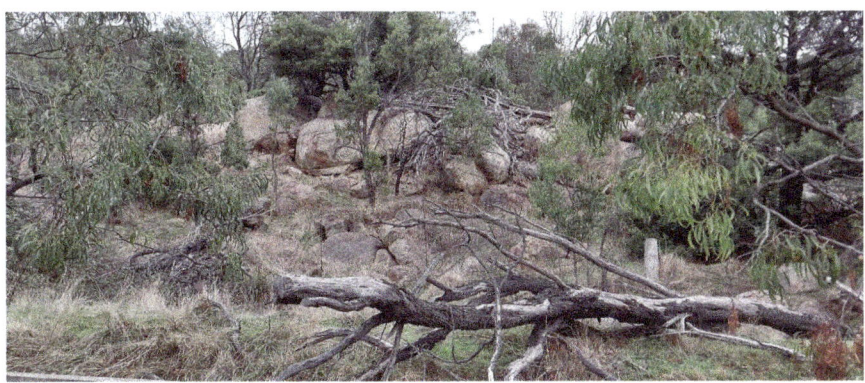

Mt Alexander Regional Park.

One of the features of the landscape on the eastern side of Mount Alexander is the rock-strewn hillslopes. It makes a scenic backdrop to the walk.

The next flume in the Wellington Flat area is not easy to see from the Access track. It appears to have been the shortest flume along this part of the walk. The granite piers have been reused to support a new concrete channel flume.

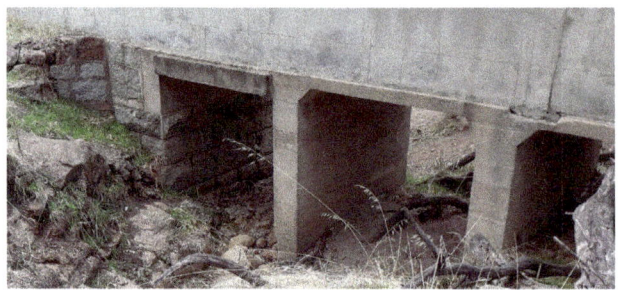

The original piers of old timber flume now reutilised.

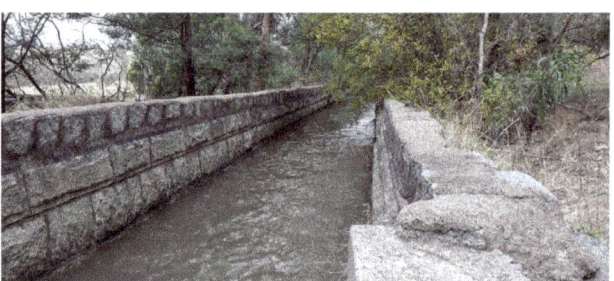

Original channel walls, Wellington Flat.

An orchard on the right (east) is one of the few remaining on this side of Mount Alexander. Once, there were many more, but fruit growing is labour intensive and the older generation of orchard owners is finding it hard to sell the idea of an often seven days a week job to a younger generation who have a lot more options available to them.[42]

A short distance past the orchard lies the car parking area on the Harcourt-Sutton Grange Road.

---

42 ABC Rural 'Apple orchards run by families dwindle in the famous apple growing region of Harcourt', 7 September 2020.

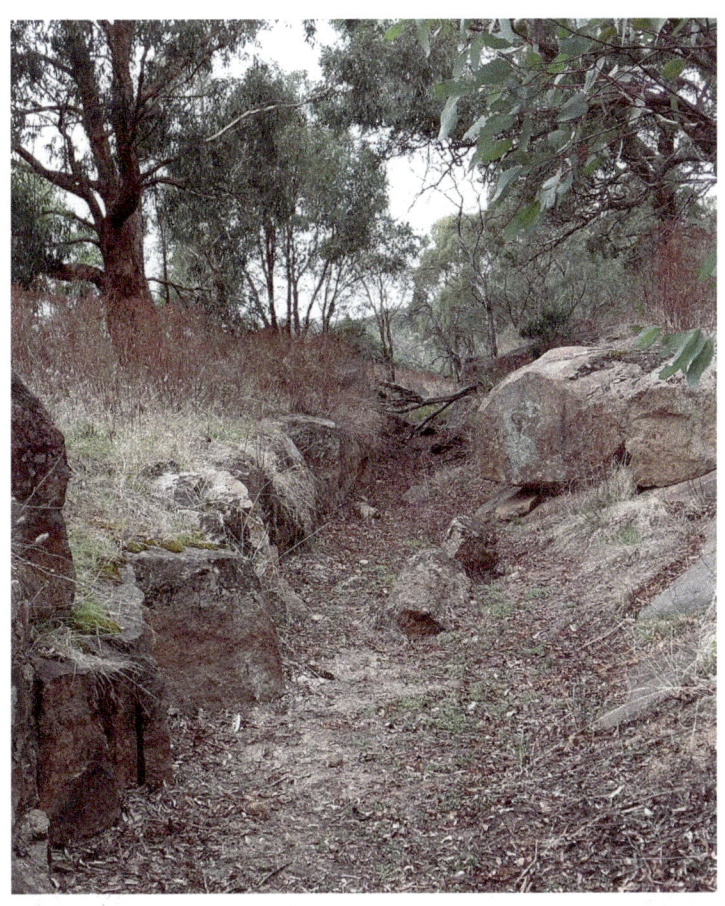
Old channel, Wellington Flat.

Harcourt-Sutton Grange Road to Youngs Lane, Harcourt North

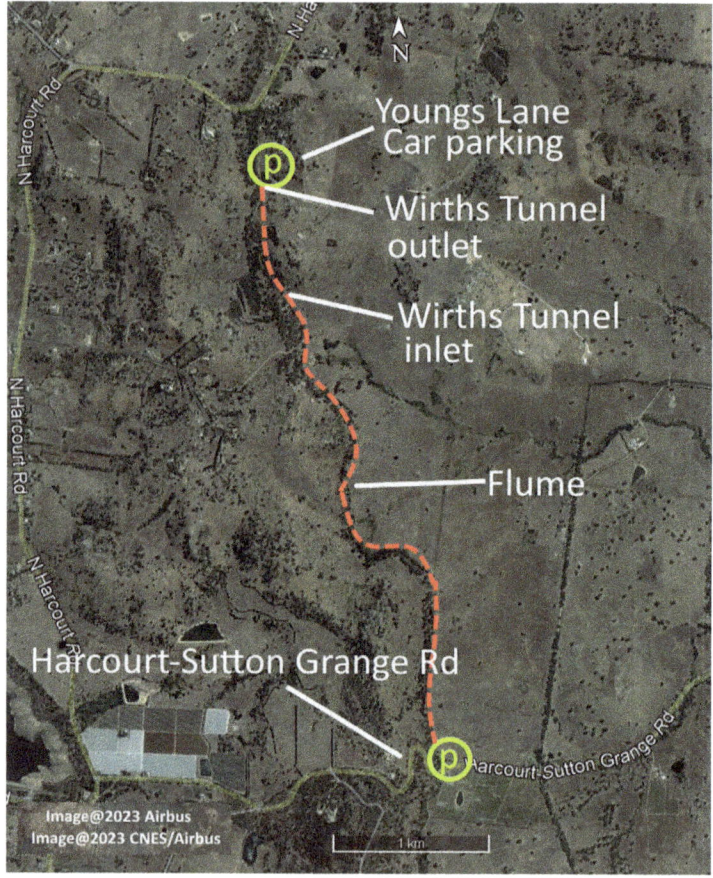

This section is part of the Leanganook Track which will take you all the way into Bendigo (but not to Crusoe Reservoir).

Again, this walk (9.6 km return) is best if you can arrange a car shuttle, one car at the parking area on the east side of the channel at its intersection with the Harcourt-Sutton Grange Road. This side track can get pretty eroded at times, with the odd muddy patch, so caution should be exercised when parking here. The other car park is in Youngs Lane off the North Harcourt Road. The intersection is tricky to see, but if you're coming from the south, it's a right turn at the bottom of the hill, just past the channel. Turn right into Youngs Lane and right again at the fork. The small car park, enough for 4 or 5 cars, is on the west side of the lane close to the channel.

If you intend to walk back the way you came, allow at least three hours for the return journey.

This is another quiet, scenic walk with a bit of a work-out climbing over the ridge that Wirths Tunnel burrows through. It starts off on a well-formed access track and heads pretty much due north.

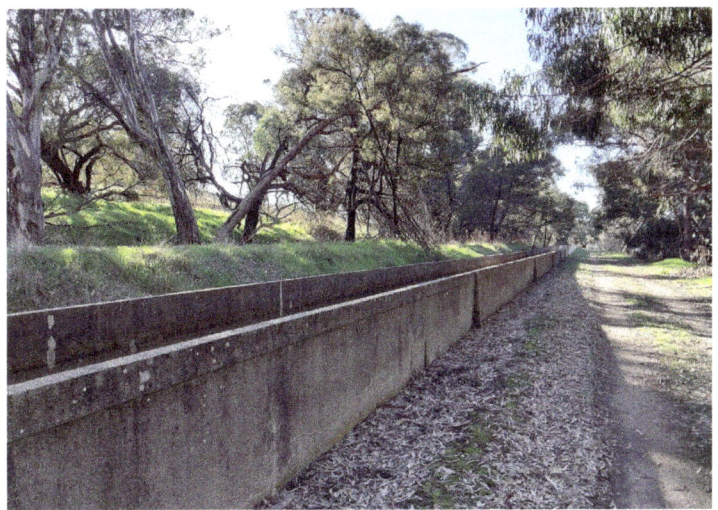

A little north of Harcourt-Sutton Grange Road, old channel far left (west).

When I walked this section in 2023 there were many sheep in the paddocks, a sign that conditions on the land had been good for farmers over the previous few years. I saw that one flock had an Alpaca guardian which kept a close watch on me as I went past. Apparently they deter foxes, chasing them and sometimes trampling them to death. As I didn't want to be trampled I kept up a brisk pace.

About two kilometres from the Harcourt-Sutton Grange Road, the track parts from the channel to descend into a gully. An interesting side trip is to keep to the channel. There's a foot track which leads to the head of a gully, yet another tributary of Axe Creek, and there's something there well worth inspecting.

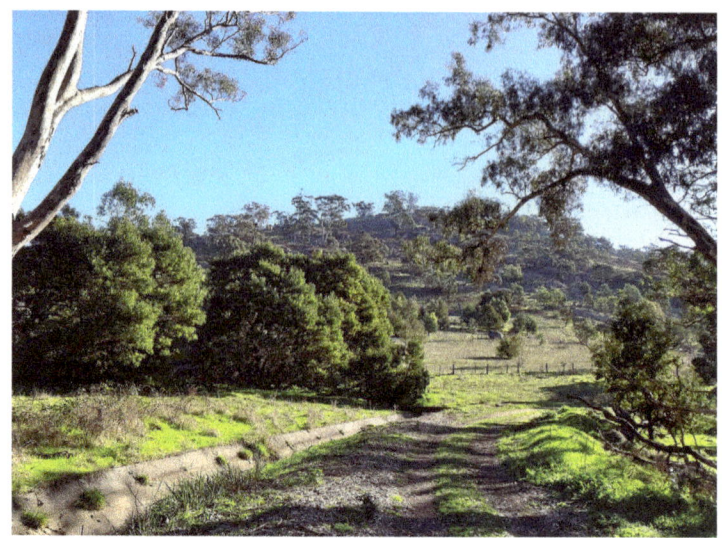
Track on the way to Wirths Tunnel.

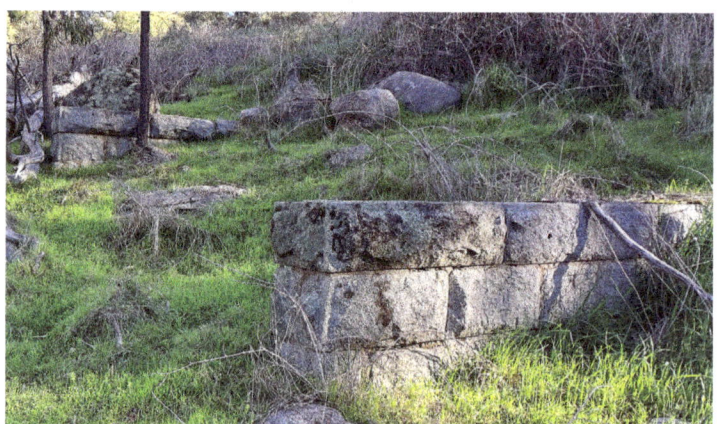
Granite footings of Flume 10.

The first items of interest are the piers of the old wooden flume which once spanned this deep gully. Quite remarkably, some of the timber sections of the flume have survived, perhaps eighty years later.

Apparently, some time before 1930, the timber flume was replaced by a concrete flume erected higher up the gully, close to the rock face. One might think that the narrowness of the gap between the rock face and flume would lead to flood debris fouling the flume.

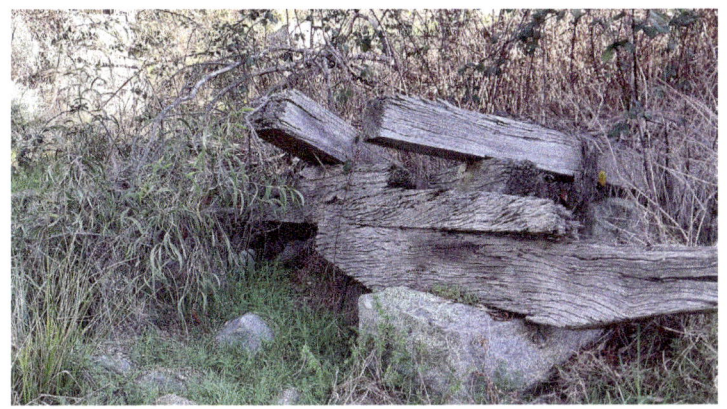

Parts of the timber undercarriage of the flume.

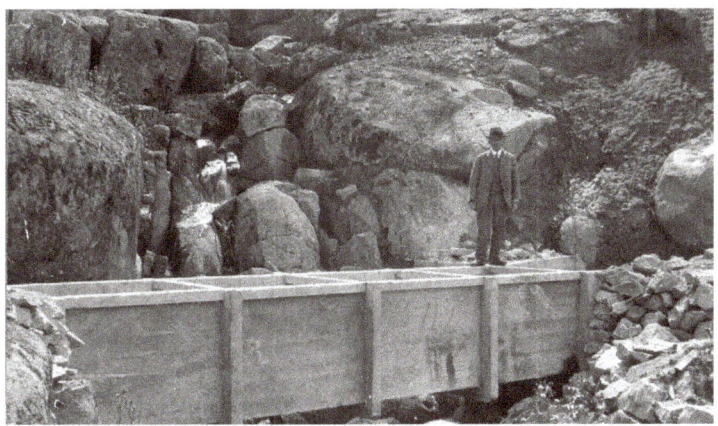

Flume 10 Axe Creek, 1930, photo SR&WSC.
Below: Present day view.

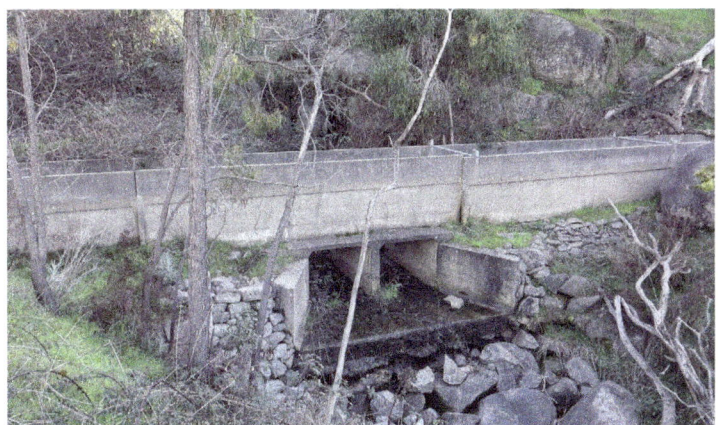

At any rate, it was decided that this wasn't the right location for this flume, and the current structure now sits a bit further out from the rocky backdrop. Sadly, the once beautiful waterfall behind is choked with blackberries.

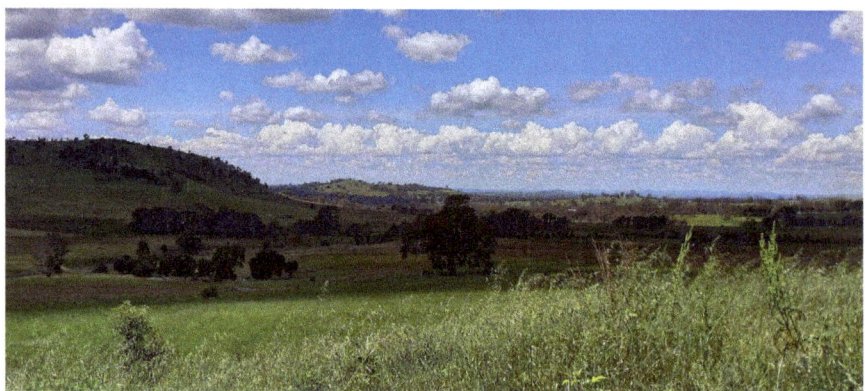

The landscape to the north-east near Wirths Tunnel.

> 'This brings us to No. 4 tunnel, at 30 miles, which is also an old work and of the same gigantic dimensions as the last. Its length is nearly half a mile, driven through granite, and it is supplied with several shafts from the summit and sides of the hill through which it passes. Its height above sea level is 1,295 feet, and the summit of the hill through which it passes 1,508 feet, the greatest depth from the crown of the hill to the tunnel being 213 feet. The entrance works to this tunnel are very large, and the material being of unstable character, the side and end slopes have been faced with turf sods, which has been done in a very neat and creditable manner, and when the grass grows on them they will present a handsome appearance. This sodding[43] was just about being finished when I was there.'
> *Bendigo Advertiser, Tuesday 20 November 1877, p. 3.*

Up ahead, the track climbs over the ridge and through freehold land. Needless to say it's important to obey the NO TRESPASS signs here and close any gate you go through. Behind the chain link barrier, there is a fenced-off tunnel work shaft. There are also spoil heaps from the tunnel's excavation.

---

43 'Sodding' is the laying of turf sections.

'On emerging from this tunnel the channel becomes much larger, its capacity having been increased in order to make it capable of receiving and conducting the large surface drainage that flows into it in this locality. It may be here mentioned that the aqueduct from this point downwards was for a long time the sole means of collecting water for the Sandhurst district, and had it not been for the foresight of Mr. Gordon in having this work completed some time ago there is good reason to believe that Sandhurst would have been on more than one occasion waterless. It is generally known, we believe, that the works at this end of the aqueduct were completed long before the connection was made with the upper portion of the channel, by which the Coliban waters were brought down.'
The Age, Thursday 3 January 1878, p. 3

Once on the other side of the ridge, the channel emerges from Wirths Tunnel and about here, on the right and very close to the channel access track, is the Youngs Lane car parking area.

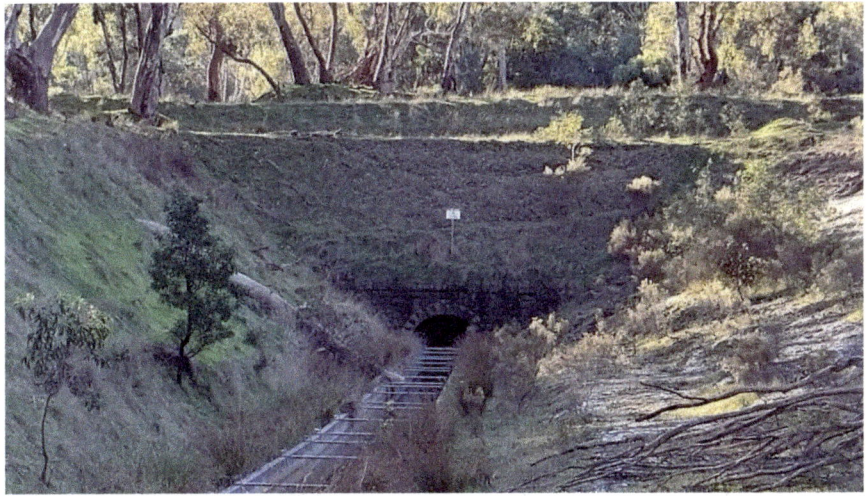

Entrance to No 4 (Wirths) Tunnel.

Youngs Lane, Harcourt North to Blossett Drive, Mandurang South

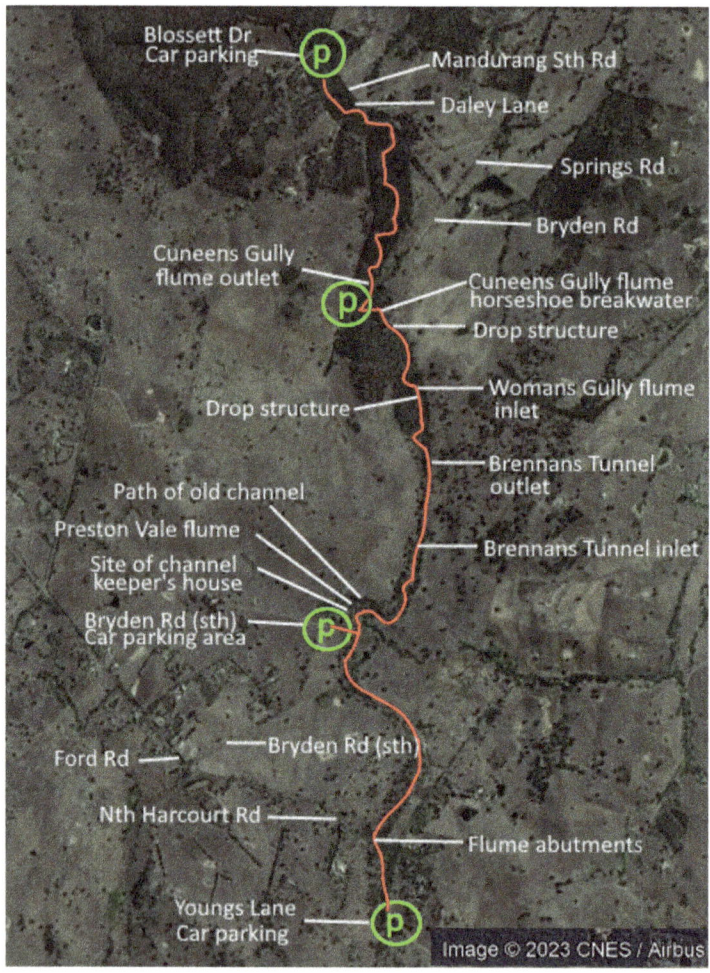

This long, but rewarding, 10.5 km walk is one of the most interesting of the Coliban Channel. It would be a long return walk if you only had one car. This is definitely best with a car shuttle.

The Youngs Lane car park is small but at a pinch could probably take about 4 or 5 cars. If coming from Harcourt, turn right immediately after the channel is crossed and then right at the next fork into Youngs Lane. A bit further on there is a small car park next to the channel reserve. If a car shuttle is arranged, walkers can leave a car at Blossett Drive or in the new parking area recently constructed in Bryden Road (see map previous page).

A shorter walk can be created by starting at the large car park off Bryden Road (south) off Ford Road.

Beginning at Youngs Lane, immediately on entering the Coliban Reserve you will see some mature fig trees next to the track. Although these trees produce copious amounts of fruit, sadly, the fruit is dry and inedible. The outlet of Wirths Tunnel is very close to the car park. Although it's unlined it has a stone retaining wall above it.

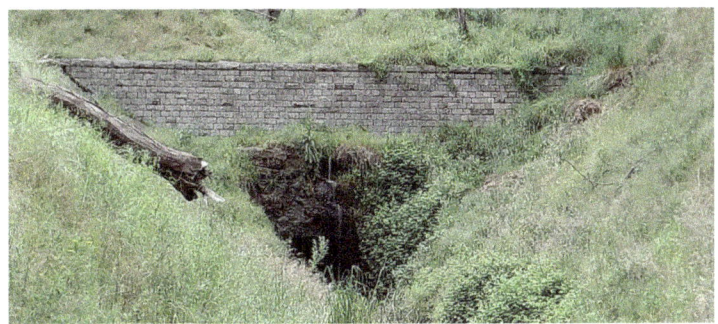

No. 4 (Wirths Tunnel) outlet.

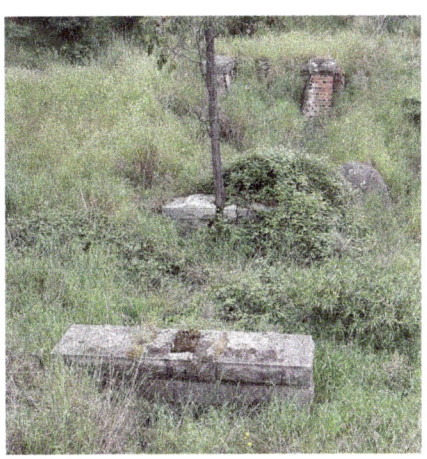

Piers and outlet abutment flume, North Harcourt Road.

After about 400 metres the North Harcourt Road must be crossed, after which, immediately to your left are the abutments of another long decommissioned flume, one of the shortest of the sixteen original flumes.

The track now runs parallel to the North Harcourt Road for some distance before heading north-west towards an area that was once known as Preston Vale.

About 1.2 km from the starting point there is a cutting and then at 1.5 km there is a marshy area where a tributary of Emu Creek

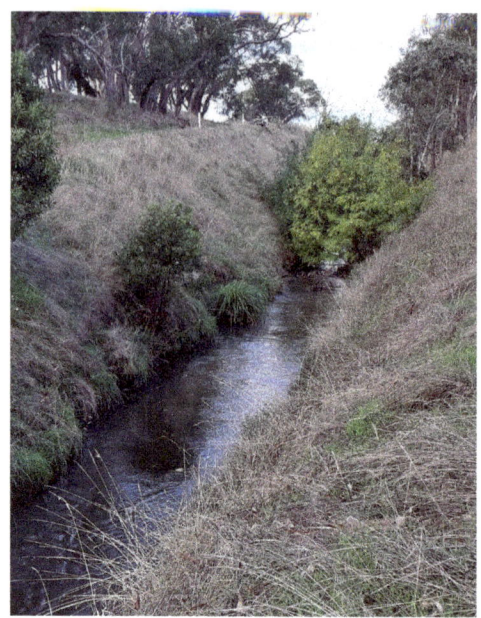 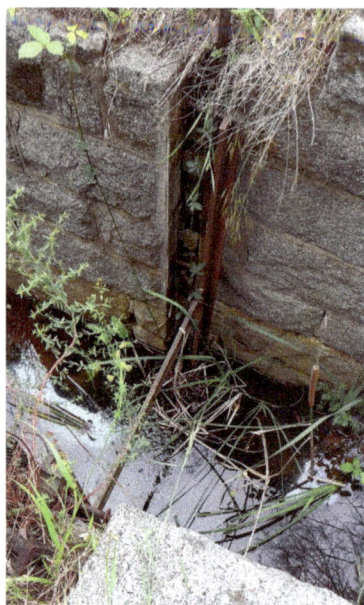

Channel at 1.5 km from Youngs Lane.   Sluice-gate, old channel.

passes under, and sometimes over, the track which has a stone floor at this point. Keep an eye out for an original metal sluice-gate built into the granite walls of the old channel here (see photo above).

At about two kilometres there is a bridge leading west over the channel to the Bryden Road (south) car park, one of the most generously proportioned parking areas along the whole channel. Next to the access track to this car park is the site of a house that once belonged to a channel keeper (later a water bailiff).[44] The old garden trees are still visible but otherwise there's very little left of the house, which, like the Sutton Grange channel keeper's house, was relocated in the 1980s, lock stock and water barrel.

The channel here has a complex history. Once a wooden flume carried the Coliban water across this tributary of Emu Creek but later, the channel was rerouted closer to the head of the creek, and the timber structure removed. This old channel is now choked with fallen timber and every kind of weed. An old sluice-gate marks the start of this disused section.

---

44 Philip Wilkin relates how the water bailiff, Jim Hodge, used to travel around the channel on horseback. Other bailiffs were Roy Furness and Earl Thomas. When the SR&WSC offered up this small parcel of land for sale, Philip's family bought and amalgamated it with their larger land holdings in the area. Philip Wilkin, *Along the Channel*, Malmsbury Historical Society, 2012.

Then, just to complicate matters, at some stage it was decided to shorten the channel by running a concrete race across the original granite piers.

There is a ledge running along the flume for those who like adventure but most will prefer safety and stick to the access track.

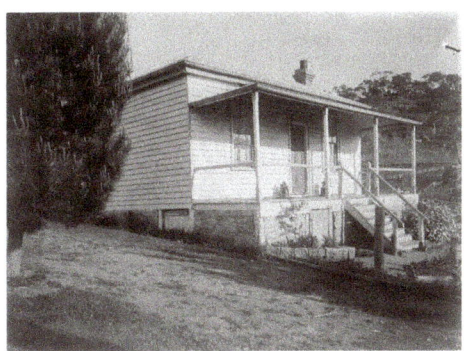 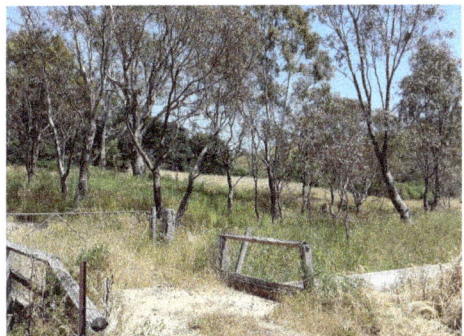

Channel keeper's house, Preston Vale. Right: House now relocated elsewhere.

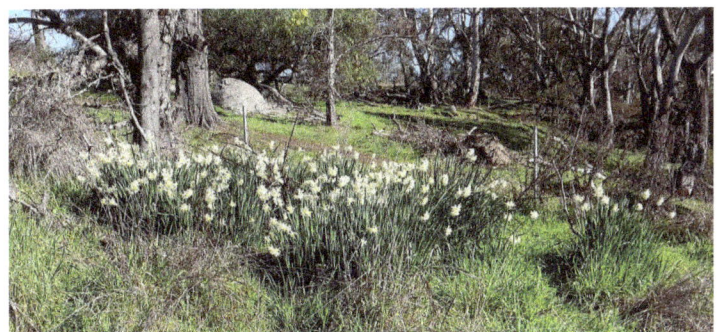

Jonquils, Preston Vale.

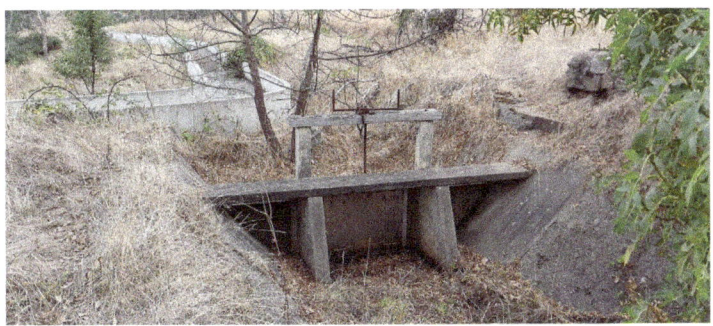

Old sluice-gate, post wooden flume channel.

'The distance from No. 4 to No. 5 tunnel is one and three-quarter miles (2.8 km). In this length there are some very fine timber flumes built by contractor Moonie on massive granite piers and abutments. There are also several works for carrying dirty drainage and flood water over the channel.'
The Age, Thursday 3 January 1878, p. 3.

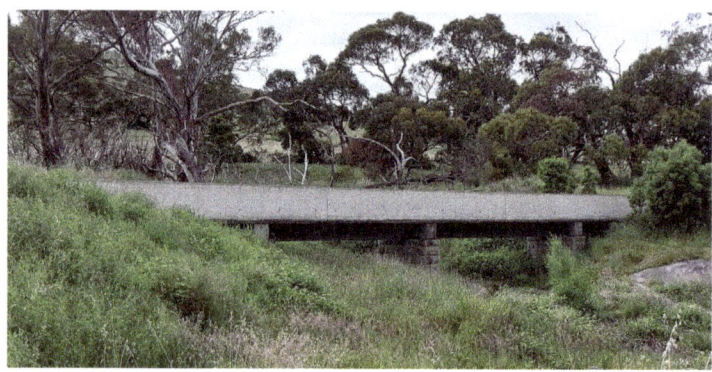

Preston Vale aqueduct or flume today.

The section from No. 4 (Wirths) Tunnel downstream to No. 7 Reservoir was the first to be built, and for some years before the completion of the entire channel, was an important catchment for the supply of water to Bendigo. However, when the headwaters of Emu Creek and Sheepwash Creek were diverted into the channel the farmers of Strathfieldsaye were up in arms. They felt robbed of the water which should have been allowed to flow down those creeks. They demanded that overshoots be installed over the channel where these creeks were crossed to allow the free flow of these streams (which were generally fed by springs in their upper reaches). When the farmers weren't complaining of creek water being diverted, they were complaining that too much water was being released from the channel into the creeks during major rain events through the sluice-gates.[45]

About 600 metres past the Preston Vale flume is the mouth of No. 5 or Brennans Tunnel, so called because Brennan was the local landowner. The entrance can barely be seen these days as blackberries have completely taken over the channel at the

---

45 *Bendigo Advertiser*, Friday 4 January 1889, p. 2.

entrance. At this point of the walk, the access track enters freehold land and so care should be taken to accede to the demands of the landholder.

'After leaving the north front of [Wirth's Tunnel], the aqueduct winds for nearly two miles on the side of hills around Preston Vale through very similar country to that of Wellington-flat, and reaches No.5 tunnel, which will make way for the water through

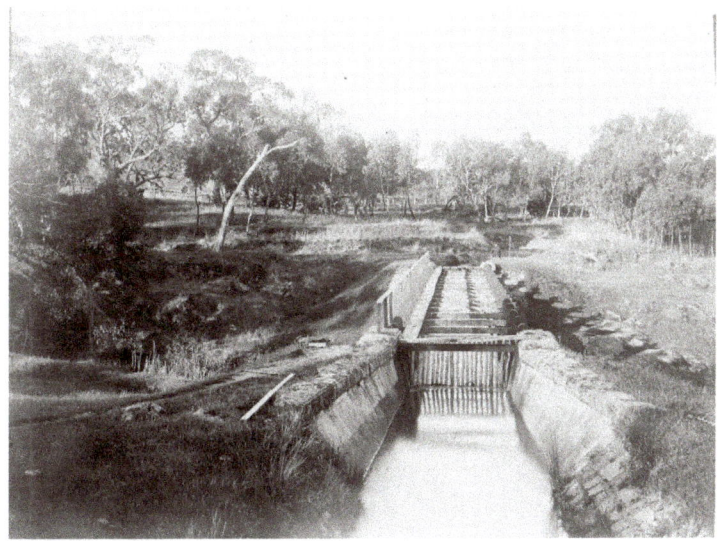

Preston Vale flume, Emu Creek, Preston Vale prior to 1920.

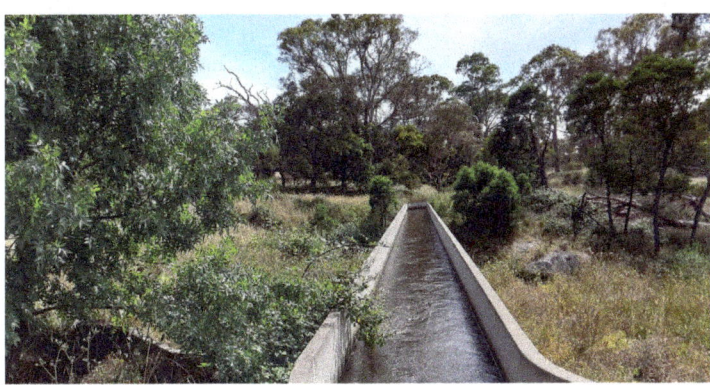

Present day view.

a spar of the same range which, at a point about ten miles to the north-west, is penetrated by the Big-hill tunnel on the Melbourne and River Murray Railway.

Messrs. Simmie and Frazer are the contractors for this work. This tunnel is in hard dense granite. ... the construction of two tunnels, Nos. 4 and 5, has enabled the engineer to dispense with about seven miles [11.3 km] of open aqueduct. ... At this work of Messrs. Simmie and Frazer, the geological character of the country suddenly changes, and the last piece of granite rock met with crops out in the aqueduct immediately north of No. 5 tunnel'.
The Australasian, Saturday 13 April 1867, p. 29.

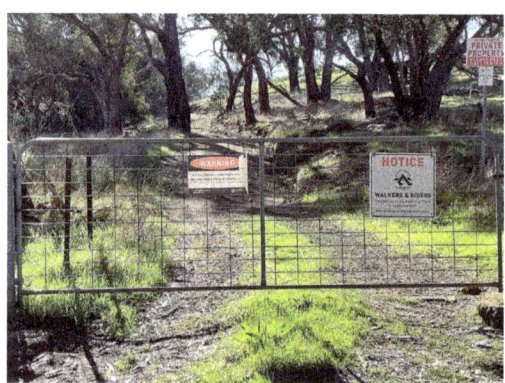

Gate on track, near No. 5 Tunnel.

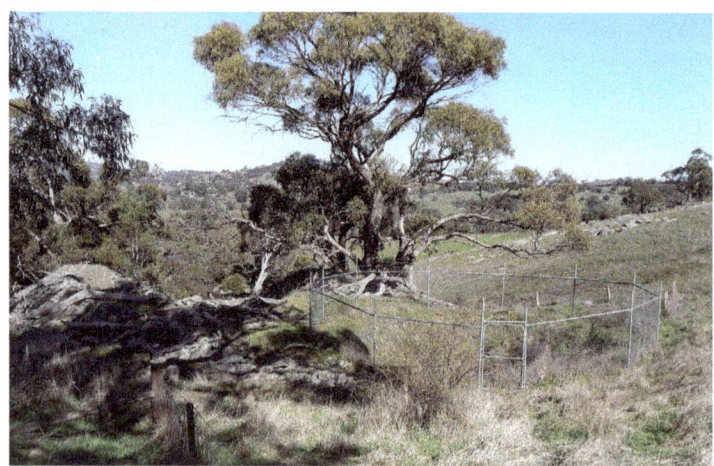

Spoil mounds and work/air shaft No 5 Tunnel.

As is the case where the track follows the underground path of No. 4 (Wirths) Tunnel, the work shaft here has been fenced off for safety reasons and the rock that had been removed during construction of the tunnel is piled up alongside the track.

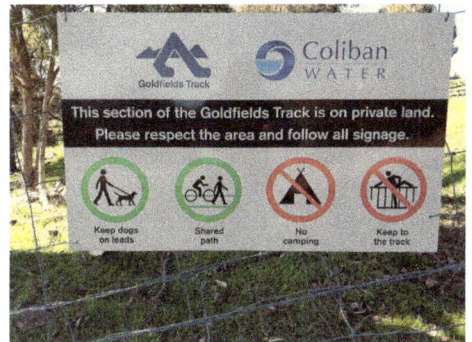

Along this part of the walk there is no shortage of signs warning walkers not to stray from the reserve.

When you reach the top of the ridge you get an expansive view of the next part of your trek along the channel.

The track now winds down the hill and rejoins the channel a little after the outlet of the No. 5 Tunnel. Both Wirths and Brennans tunnels are unlined and were built when economy was needed in order to finish the Coliban Water Scheme, the budget of which had been well and truly blown.

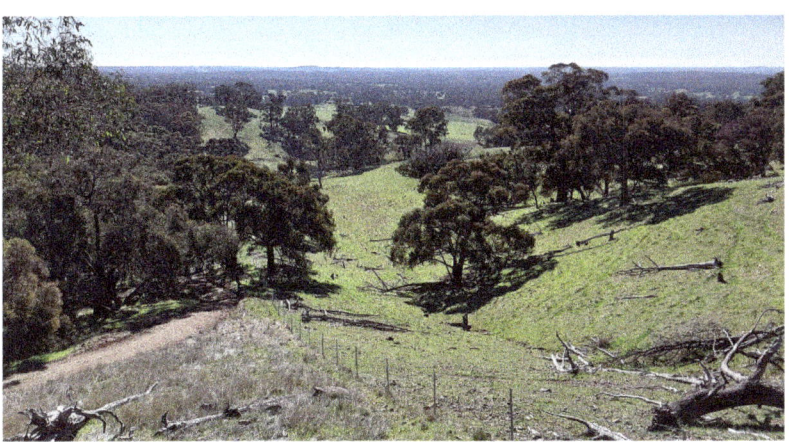

View towards Bendigo from No. 5 Tunnel ridge.

If there's a starring attraction along the Coliban Channel it's the engineering marvels between the outlet of the No. 5 tunnel and Bryden Road (once known as Springs Road). That they're a well kept secret is probably due to there being no easy access to them, at least for the casual tourist. Springs Road was once the main route between Harcourt North and localities east of Bendigo such as Strathfieldsaye and Axedale. This can be seen by the odd angle Springs Road makes when it meets Sedgwick Road. In the not too distant past, a local landowner blocked off access to through traffic (which once travelled up Springs Road from a point

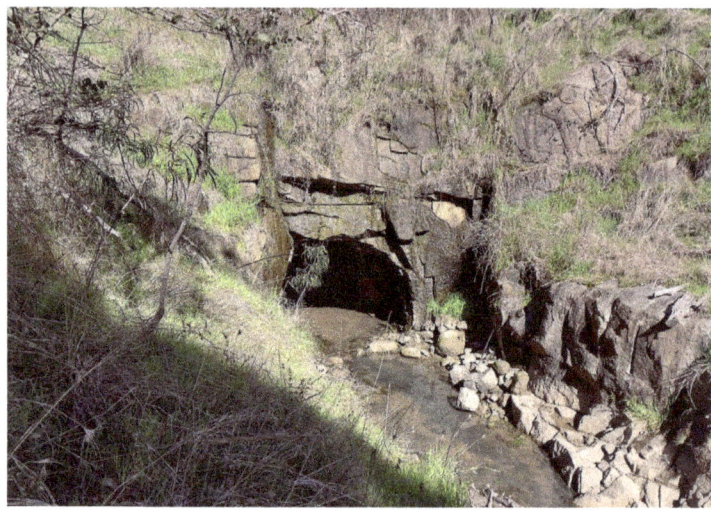

No. 5 (Brennans) Tunnel outlet.

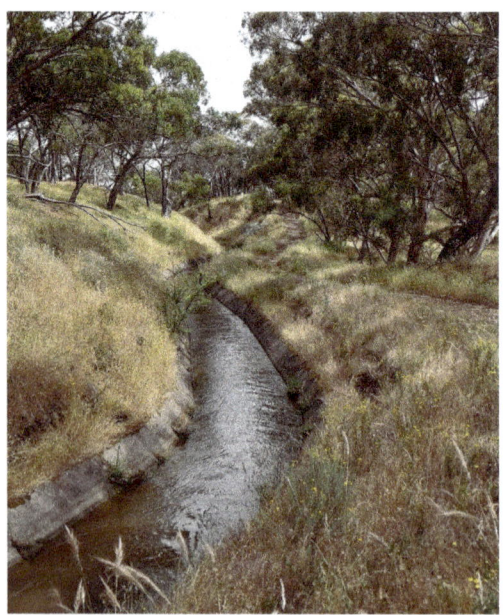

Channel before the drop structures.

near the intersection of Ford and North Harcourt Roads).[46] The reason given was that illegal shooters and other mischief makers were a danger to roaming stock. It continues the trend of farmers blocking access to old rights of way which bisect their land.

> 'After passing through No. 5 tunnel, which is a little over a quarter of a mile long, at 1,284 feet above sea level, and the summit of the hill through which it passes 1,472 feet, we come to section 5 (the last), which, with section 4, up to Crusoe Gully Reservoir has been made since 1873. ... The fall is about 5 feet per mile, with several large drops at intervals, available when required for motive powers, should machinery be erected close by.
>
> Although these works have been in use for years, to all appearances they were in perfect order, although some slight repairs and extension of walling are evidently required; but this is in parts that have not been quite finished, particularly in the floors of the drops, which require cementing in places. In conclusion of my general description, I understand that the first sections of the channel are designed to carry up to ten million gallons per day'.
>
> *Bendigo Advertiser, Tuesday 20 November 1877, p. 3.*

> 'A few chains distant from the No. 5 tunnel the character of the Country changes from granite to schist.[47] A drop cutting is now entered. It passes through a sandstone spur, on the margin of which the water flows over a drop of 28 feet [8.5 m] into a large brick tank, from which it emerges and is conducted over a valley by a large timber flume 250 feet [76.2 m] long, and built on piles. The conduit then contours along steep sideling country for about half a mile [804 m], when another drop similar to the last is encountered. It is divided, however, into two lengths, making a total fall of eighty-six feet [26.2 m]. This, like the last, also falls into a very fine brick tank, surmounted with a well-finished

---

46 In descriptions of the channel from the 1870s I can find no mention of North Harcourt Road (east of Ford Road), which indicates that it might not have been constructed at that time.

47 Schist is a coarse-grained metamorphic rock which consists of layers of different minerals and can be split into thin irregular plates ref. Oxford Dictionary .

coping. In the centre of this tank a horse-shoe wall is built. This wall is fitted with ports, through which the water flows into the down-stream end of the tank, from whence it emerges into a flume, by which it is carried across a road and Cuneen's Gully'
The Age, Thursday 3 January 1878, p. 3.

As you climb a hill, at least when the water is running in the channel, you gradually become aware of the roar of a waterfall and at the top of the rise, to your left is a lookout (complete with a monstrous meat ant nest, so it pays to be nimble on your feet!). Here you can see a stream of water pouring over the edge in a vertical sheet to race down a long chute. This is the first of two similar structures in this area.

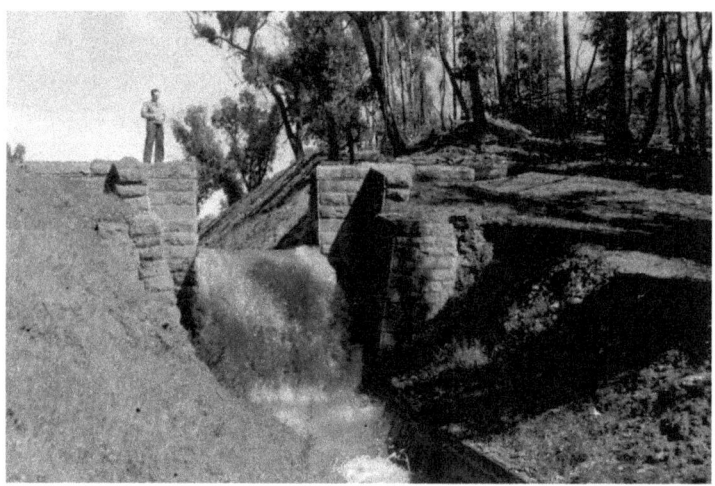

Womans Gully chute, 1940, SR&WSC.

'The flumes on this section, four in number, like the others, are built of redgum timber framings and deal troughs, the former resting on granite ashlar piers, and the two latter [Womans and Cuneens gullies flumes] on red-gum piles. Those troughs, like the channel, are larger, being about 5 feet wide by 3 feet in depth.

At Woman's[48] and Cuneen's gullies, there are two drops, the former being 30 feet [9.1 m] deep, and the latter about 80 feet [24.4 m]. At the head of each the drop is nearly vertical for 12

---

48 According to Wilkin, p. 59 the local name for this gully was Old Womans Gully.

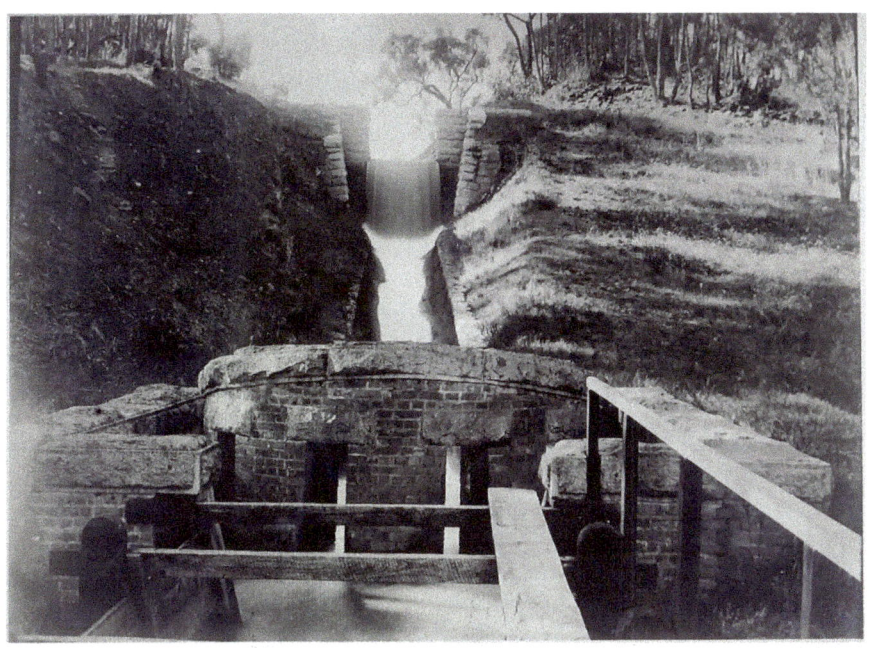

Womans Gully chute, looking south prior to ca 1920. Below: Present day view.

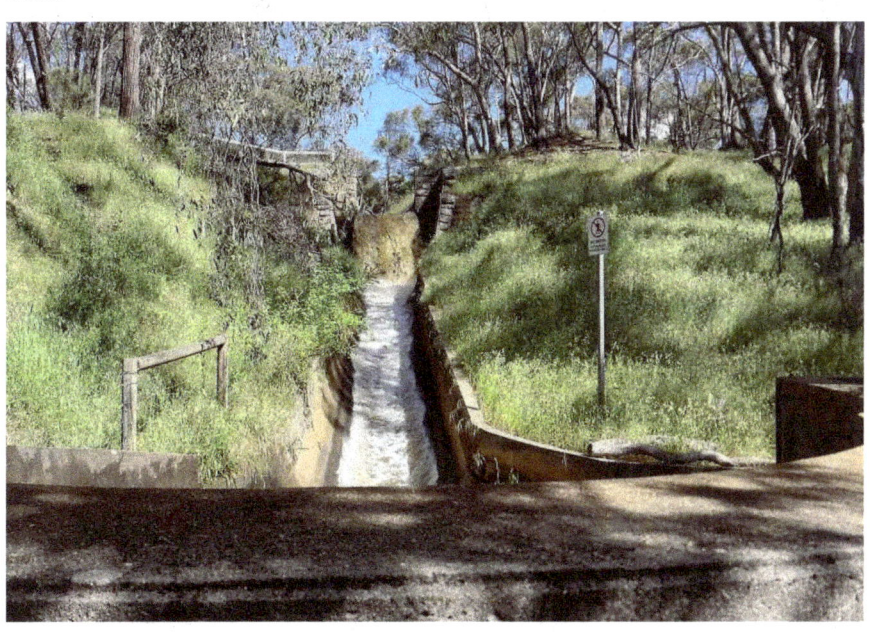

feet, after which the water flows down an incline plane into large tanks with horseshoe breakwaters,[49] and from thence to the flumes, which convey it across the gullies. Along the open channel there are side sluice-gates, waste weirs, bridges, overshoots, etc., which all bear the stamp of good workmanship.'
Bendigo Advertiser, Tuesday 20 November 1877, p. 3.

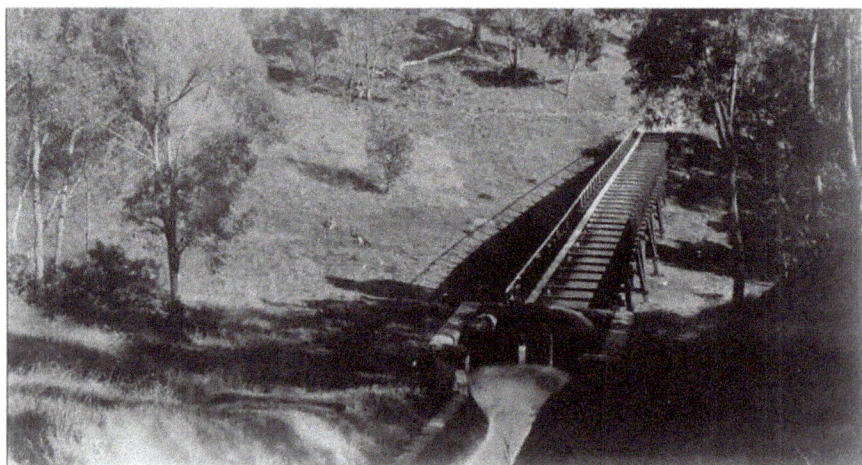

Womans Gully flume looking north. Below: Present day view.

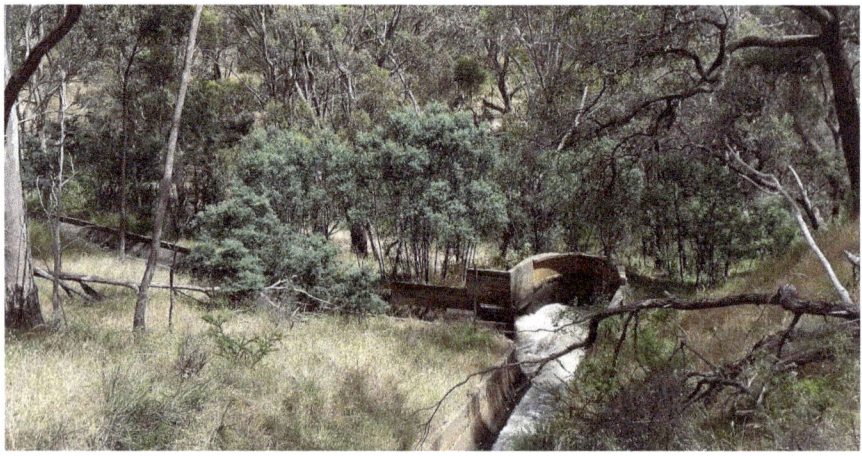

---

49 These structures are designed to absorb and dissipate the energy of rapidly flowing water. They are now generally called dissipators.

As you descend the track you will see that the old horseshoe breakwater has been modified. Instead of the water flowing through the ports in the breakwater, the channel has been rerouted sideways, not only to cut the rate at which the water descends, but to do away with the wooden flume (which surely required continual maintenance).

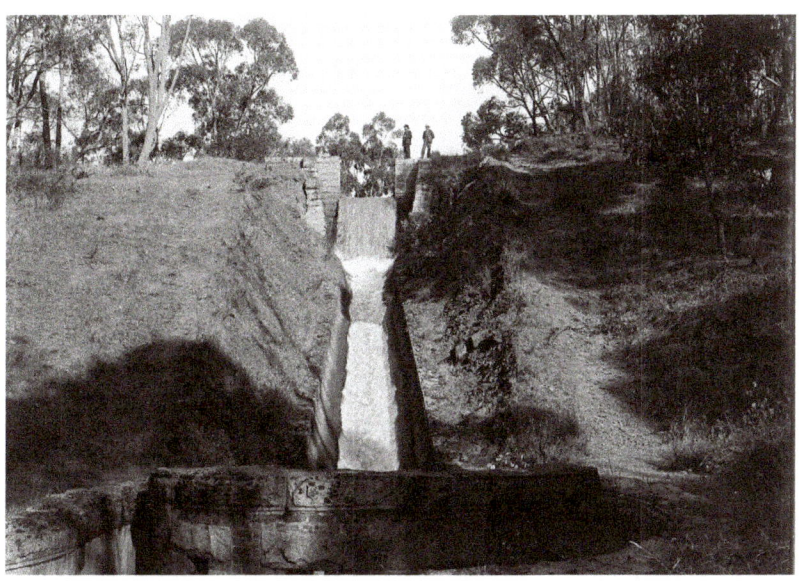

Cuneens Gully Chute, 1900, Rural Water Corporation Collection. Below: Present day view.

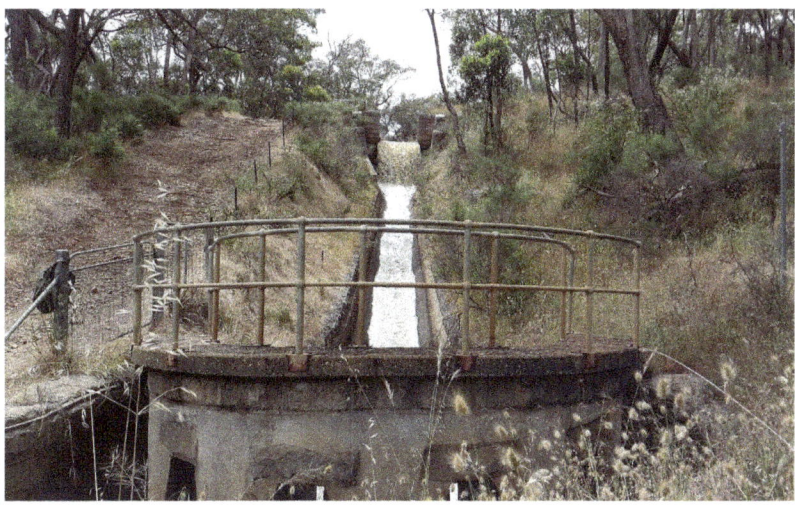

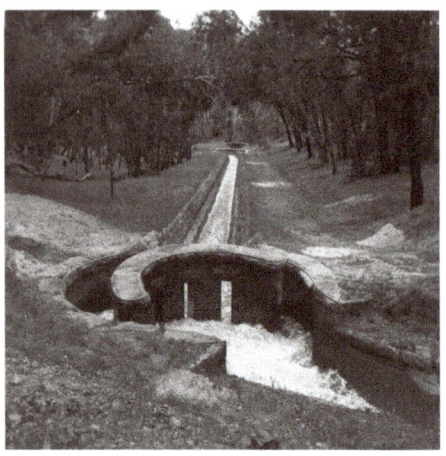
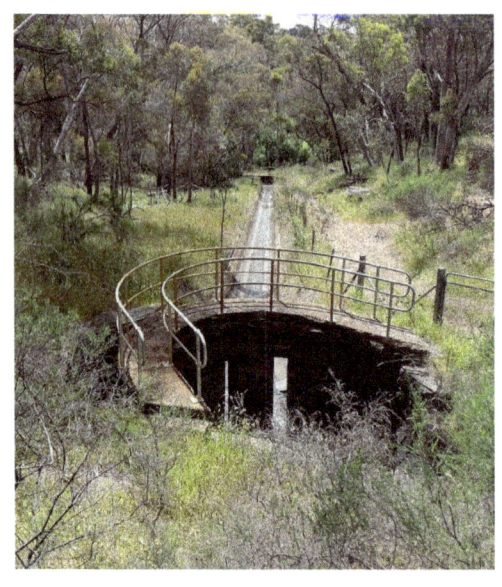

Cuneens Gully chute (decommissioned horseshoe breakwater in distance). Right: Present day view.

The track passes below the horseshoe breakwater at Womans Gully and loops around, following the path of the more recently constructed channel.

Within a short distance, as the track rises again, the noise of another waterfall can be heard. This structure is the even more spectacular Cuneens Gully drop chute. Here there are two breakwaters or dissipators, although only one is still in use.

There is now a locked gate barring access to the walkway on top of the breakwater. This is probably due to the deteriorating quality of the concrete top. It's certainly a thrilling sight watching the water cascade down the long chute.

As in the case of the previous Womans Gully drop chute and flume, the old wooden flume has been removed and a concrete race now loops around closer to the head of the gully. This has meant that the lowest horseshoe breakwater has been isolated from the channel. It can be seen overlooking Bryden Road (see bottom photo next page).

Recently, Bryden Road (old Springs Road)[50] was graded and a parking area created near a new visitor shelter. While being a

---

50 Springs Road is the old name of the road which ran between the North Harcourt Road, north to Sedgwick Road. It now only refers to that section between Sedgwick Road and South Mandurang Road. The old southern section, no longer a through road, is now known as Bryden Road.

welcome development, the road works have destroyed what may well have been a remnant of early rural road construction (see page 149).

It's possible to follow the Channel itself rather than the access track after it crosses Bryden Road, but it requires a bit of off-track navigation (and maybe the risk of damp feet when jumping over the nascent Emu Creek).

And now for the final 2.5 km to Blossett Drive where you might have left a car. If returning to Youngs Lane you might choose to turn around at this point. If you're doing a two-day

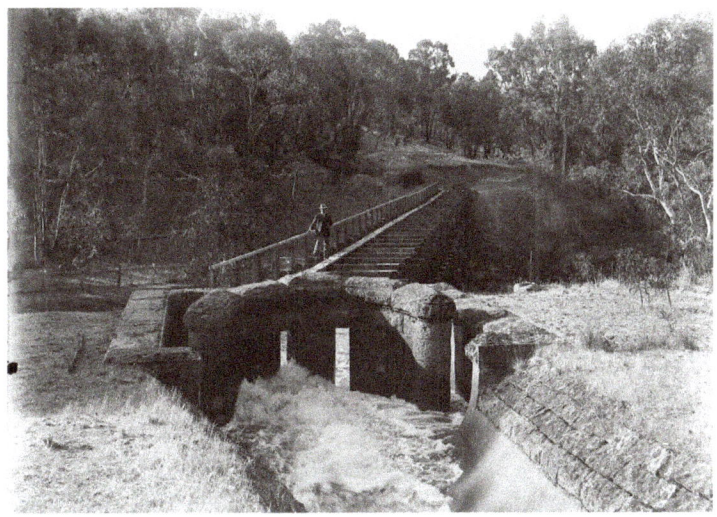

Cuneens Gully horseshoe breakwater and Bryden Road (Springs Road) flume, looking north, 1900. Below: Present day view.

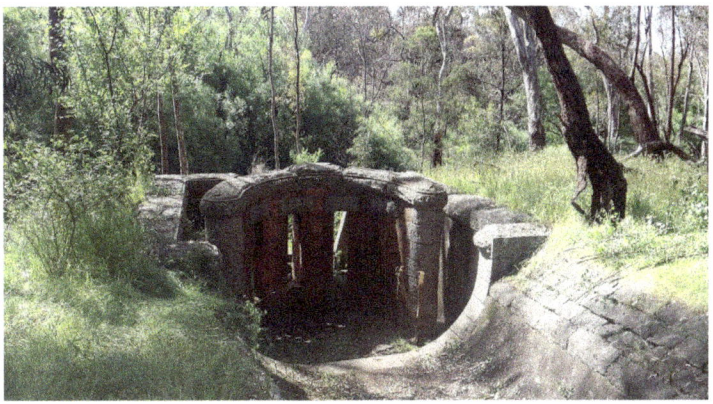

walk you might head for your overnight camp site at the Goom Gooruduron-Yeran Campground (403 Mandurang South Road). In that case, hopefully, there'll be water in the untreated rainwater tank close to the junction of the Leanganook Track and the channel access track.

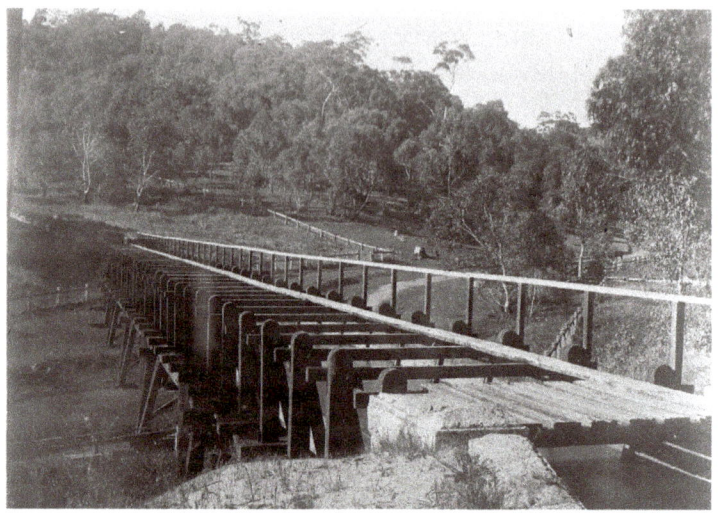

Cuneens Gully flume outlet, looking north. Below: Present day view.

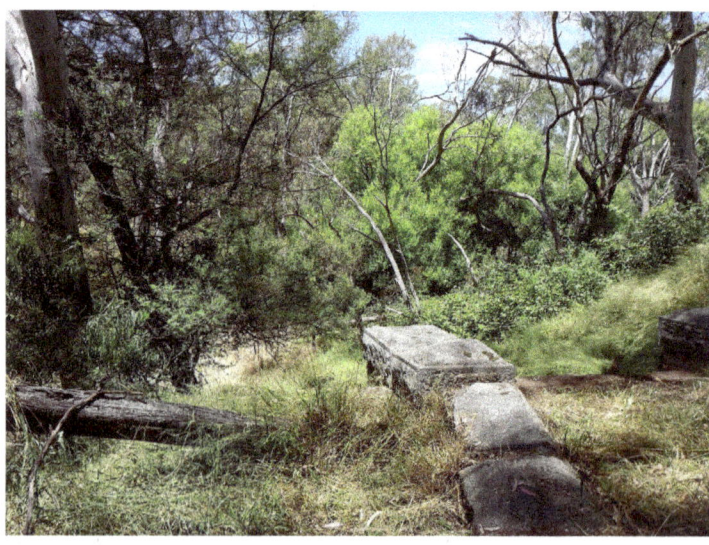

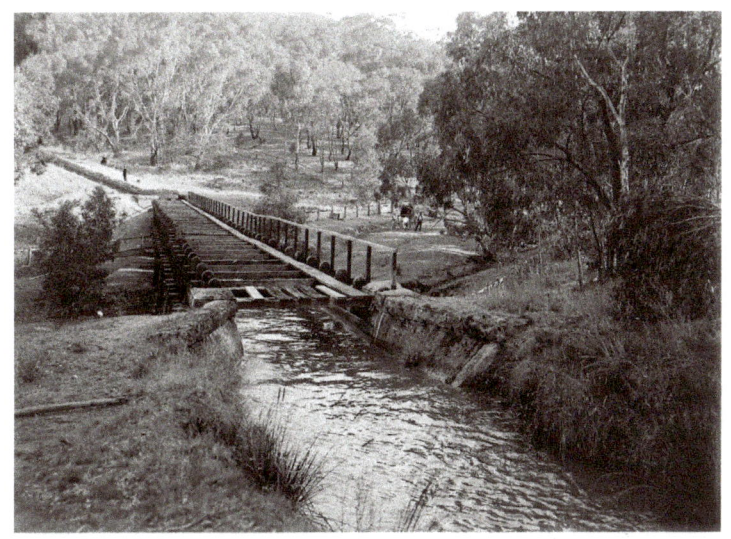

Another view of Cuneens Gully flume prior to 1930.

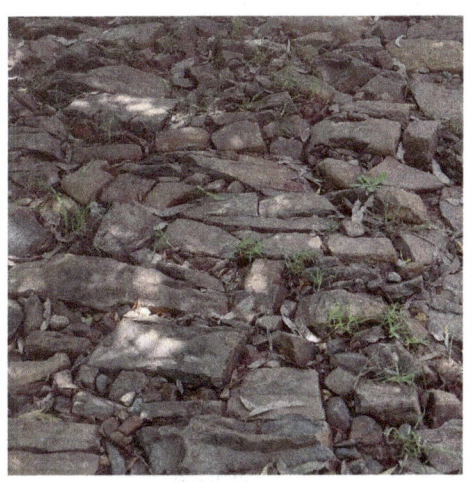 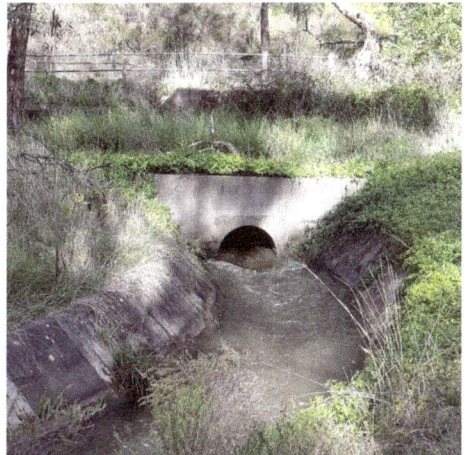

Bryden Road (before recent grading).   *Culvert under Bryden Road.*

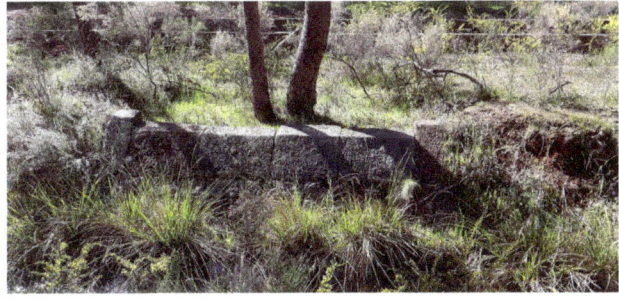

Waste weir near Daley Lane, old channel. (For a likely explanation for this structure see page 155.)

The interesting channel structures near Bryden Road have long attracted sightseers, yet little had been done to cater for them. Thankfully, in late 2023, public requests to improve facilities finally bore fruit. The creation of a parking area and a visitor shelter alongside the Leanganook Track may well lead to an increase in the number of tourists visiting this area. Because of likely visitor demand for the limited number of car spaces here, this walk ends, and the next walk starts, at Blossett Drive.

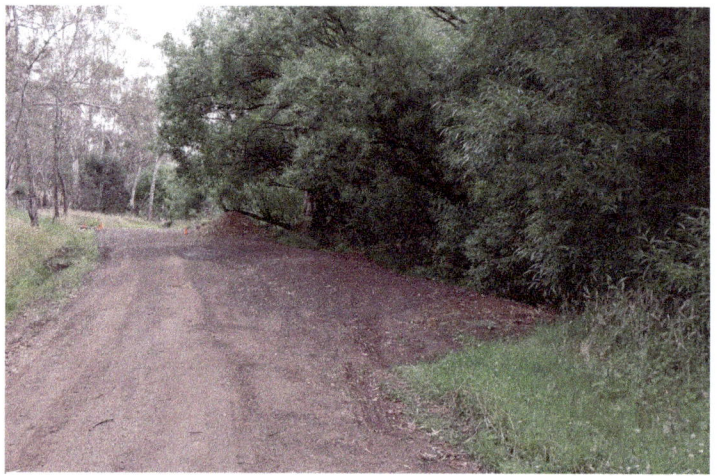

New car parking area, Bryden Road.

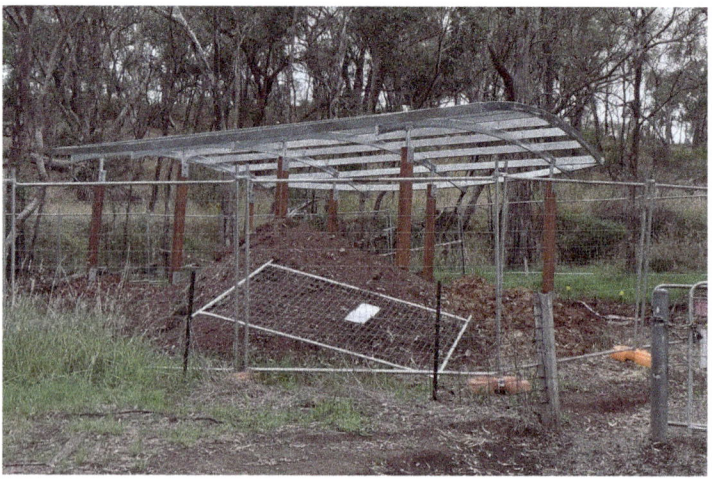

Visitor shelter under construction, Bryden Road.

Blossett Drive to Harpers Road

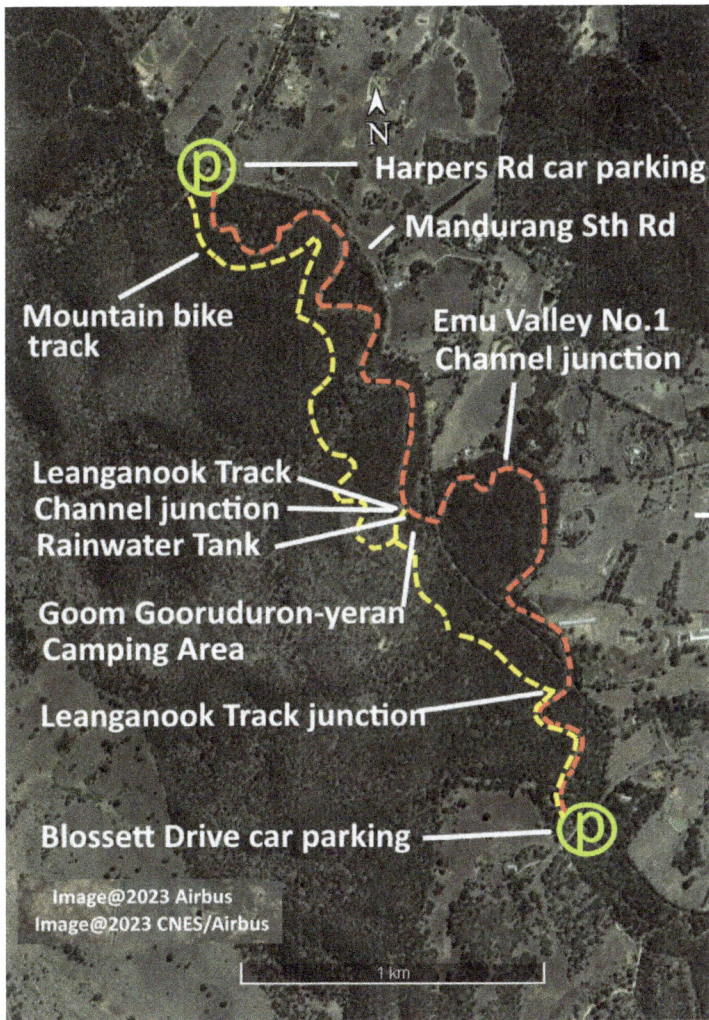

This walk is about 8.5 km return. There is a car parking area in Blossett Drive near the channel. There is ample car parking at Harpers Road near the gate marking the entrance to the Greater Bendigo National Park.

An option for those returning to their car from Harpers Road is to walk along a mountain bike track which meanders inside the

Greater Bendigo National Park. But be warned, dirt bikes have taken to using it as well, leading to the erosion of the track.

Once through the gate at Blossett Drive walking is straightforward and easy along the well maintained access track.

Within about 700 metres, the Leanganook track heads off over the channel and into the National Park. Apparently this was done to avoid having to cross the Mandurang South Road twice,[51] but for those wishing to follow the channel, there is no other option than to look right, left and right again and cross the road.

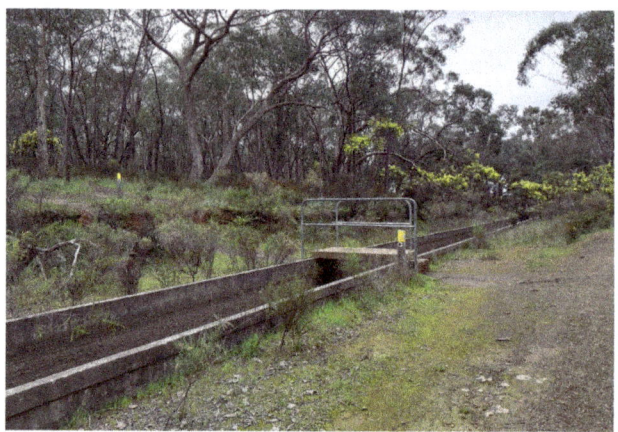

Junction of Leanganook Track and channel access track.

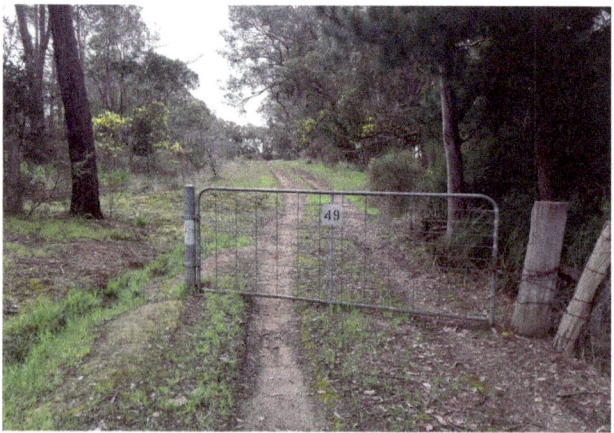

Gate 49, east side Mandurang South Road.

---

51 Wilkin, p. 65.

Within a short distance there is a large egg farm to your right. If it's a nice day, a thousand or so chickens will race up to the fence hoping you might say hello and offer a handful of grain. As you pass you will notice a cage out in the open with a solar panel on top. This is a fox trap. According to workers there, a few foxes continue to break in with evil intentions.

Along this section, the channel becomes wider and begins to resemble a large creek. In the early years, quite a few side streams were captured by the channel, and so the channel had to be large enough to handle the additional flow.

About 750 metres past the chicken farm the Emu Valley No. 1 channel junction is met. This side channel might look modest at

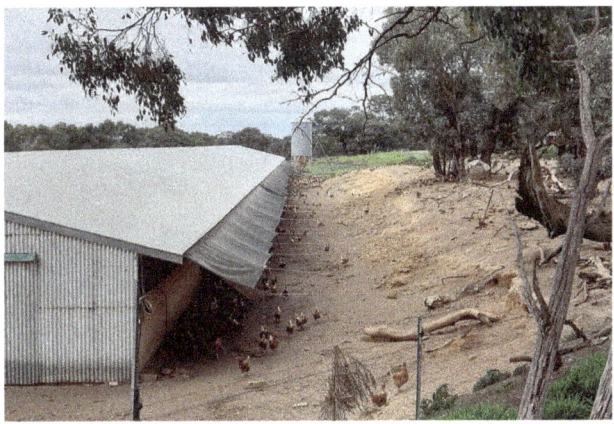
Free range egg farm.

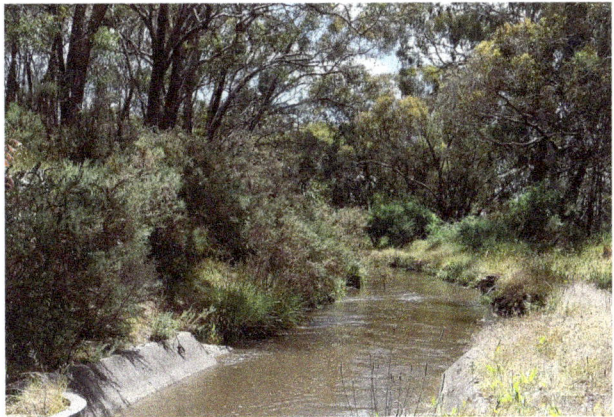
Channel near egg farm.

this point, but it winds its way many kilometres to the east, to Sedgwick, Strathfieldsaye and beyond.

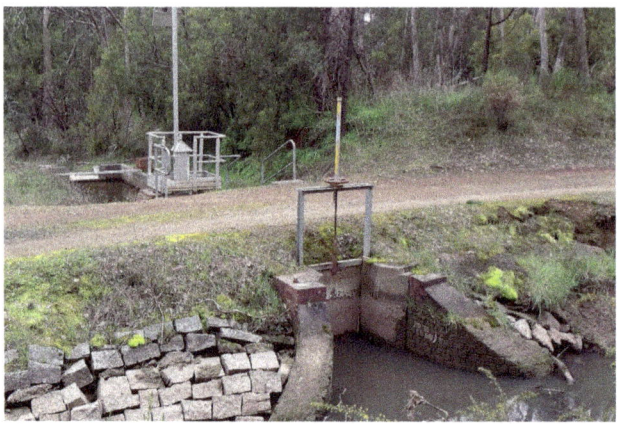

Emu Valley No. 1 Channel junction.

'Strathfieldsaye farmers who were in Bendigo on Saturday were jubilant on account of the prospects of an improved water supply from the old Emu Valley channel which was a short time ago thrown open for irrigation purposes. The channel, which branches off the Coliban race about half a mile[52] [804 m] from the flumings at The Springs,[53] has been in the hands of the Government for the past two years. But it was not until recently that steps were taken to utilise it for diverting the water on to the cultivated lands around the Strathfieldsaye and Mandurang districts. ... The water has only been available for about three weeks, and the beneficial results, especially to the fruit trees, are regarded as wonderful. ... The channel extends as far as Mr

---

52 This measurement is incorrect. As the crow flies, the distance from the 'flumings at The Springs' to the present day Emu Valley No.1 Channel junction is about 2.8 km (over 1.7 miles). Construction of the channel began in May 1889 and was administered by the Emu Valley Irrigation and Water Supply Trust until it was wound up in 1898 when the spread of phylloxera in the region led to a dramatic decrease in demand for water (and the ability to pay it) from the young wine industry.

53 Apparently, 'The Springs' (presumably at the head of Emu Creek and hence the name of the road) was a popular picnic spot at the time.

Reid's property, a little over a mile from the Shire Hall,[54] and when it is got into proper working order between 50 and 60 landholders will be able to irrigate.'
Bendigo Advertiser, Monday 19 February 1906, p. 5.

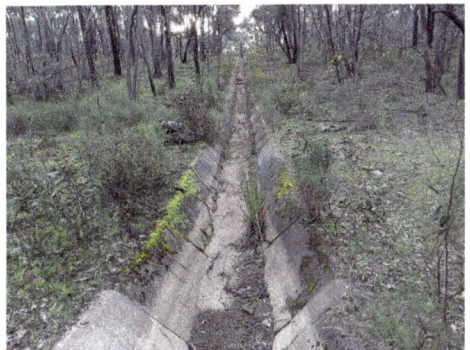

Emu Valley No. 1 Channel, Hogans Road.

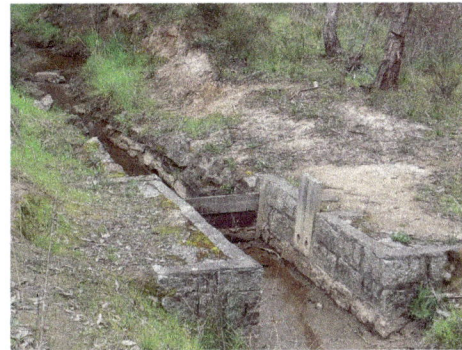

Emu Valley No. 2 Channel, Sedgwick.

Along the old superseded Coliban channel there are interesting structures whose purpose seems unclear. These stone structures appear to be waste weirs (now stormwater overpours).[55] When the channel overflows during a severe rain event, rather than allow the floodwaters to overflow the earthen banks and possibly cause their erosion or collapse, weirs were built into the channel walls to take the strain. These structures only occur on one side of the channel and don't appear to be the foundations of overshoots.

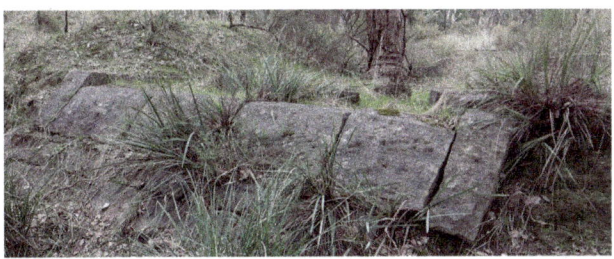

Granite waste weir.

---

54 The Strathfieldsaye Shire Hall in Strathfieldsaye Road still survives relatively unaltered.

55 'Granite waste weirs are also provided at proper distances on the lower side to carry off the surface storm-waters when the channel becomes too full for its safety, and, as a rule, discharge themselves into natural creeks.' *The Bendigo Advertiser*, 20 November 1877, p. 2.

In 250 metres the Mandurang South Road is crossed again. Once across the road the Leanganook track is encountered once more. Near here there is a water tank, full, hopefully, of unfiltered rainwater. The tap is spring loaded so filling a bucket for ablutions is a job for those with plenty of patience.

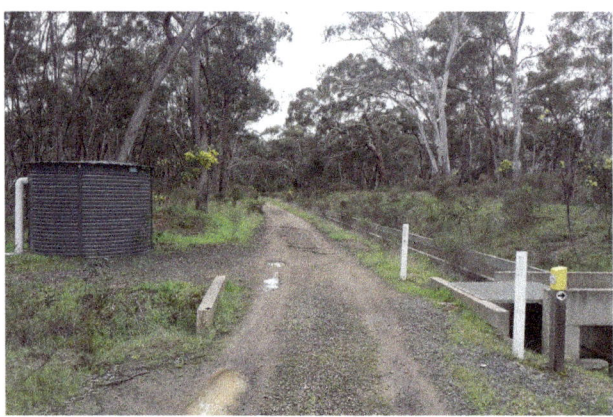

Rainwater tank and Leanganook Track junction.

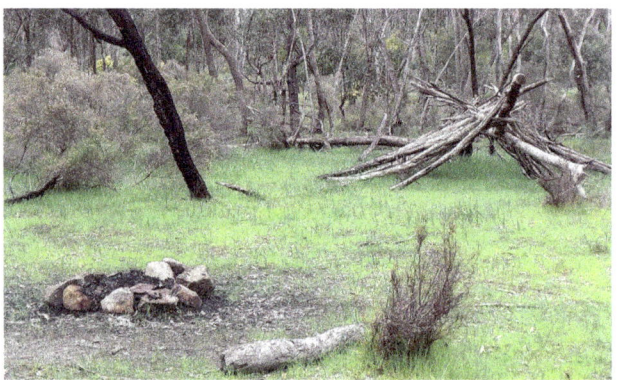

Goom Gooruduron-yeran Campground.

For those hikers undertaking a two day walk, Goom Gooruduron-yeran Campground is a short walk back down the Leanganook track, but don't expect too much in the way of comfort, such as a toilet block.

Back on the Leanganook track, across the other side of the concrete race you will catch glimpses of the old decommissioned channel. Unfortunately, for most walkers the old historic features which still adorn the old channel will be out of reach and sight.

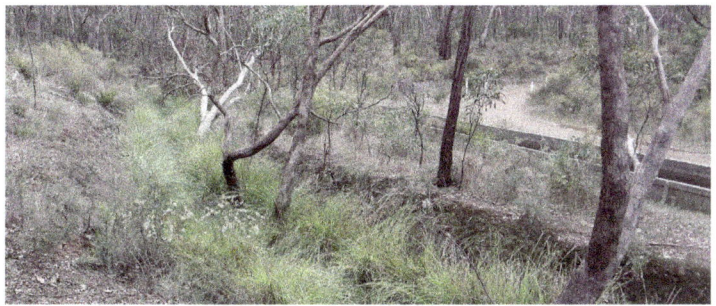

The original channel on the left.

Not far from Harpers Road there is a brick structure on the banks of the channel which is probably an old sluice-gate, which, when opened, would have allowed water to pour into the gully in the background – draining water away and allowing maintenance to be done on the channel further downstream. The flow from Malmsbury would have been halted prior to this happening.

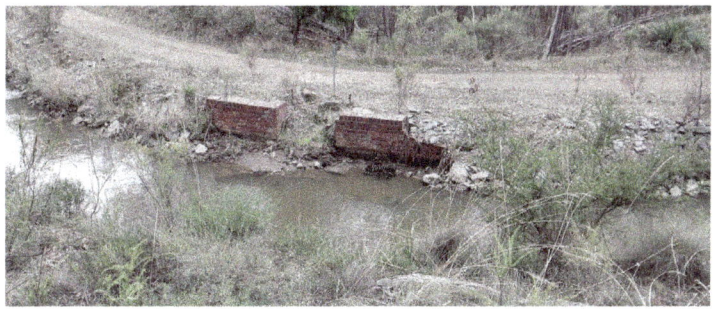

Ruins of old sluice-gate.

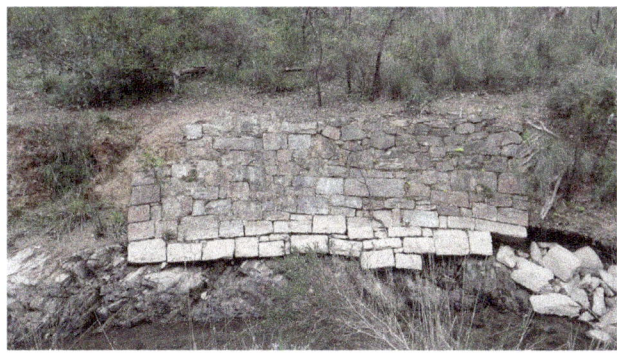

Stormwater runoff under low flow conditions.

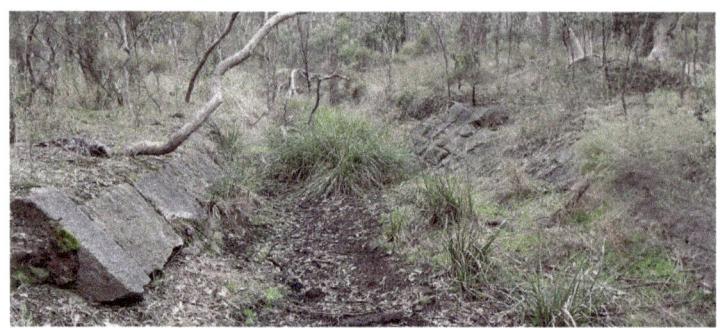

Old channel near Harpers Road. Note, another granite waste weir on the downslope side (looking south in this photo).

Another feature of the channel along this section is the reinforced stone-lined stormwater runoff ramps designed to prevent the erosion of the channel sides by incoming floodwaters.

It's now not far to Harpers Road. The car parking area is down a short section of track to your right (east). Somebody has been very creative with a fence post here. Perhaps an attempt at levity as an antidote to the recurring vandalising of gates by those insisting on continued vehicle access to the Greater Bendigo National Park.

For those returning to Blossett Drive, an alternative route is to follow the mountain bike track to the west of the channel. It's easy to find the start of the track back because the gate here is usually lying flat on the ground.

Anyone who has walked mountain bike trails knows that one needs to have plenty of patience and be willing to take the long way home as the track meanders along.

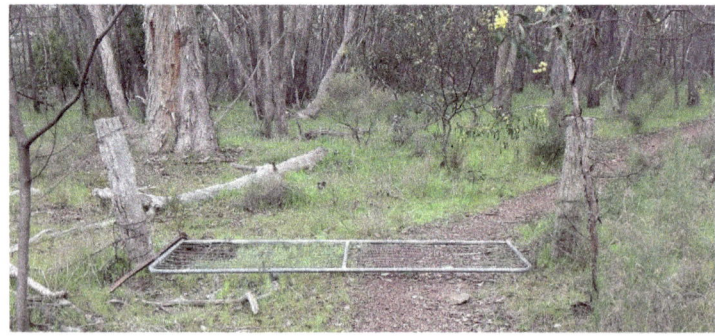

Entry to mountain bike trail.

Finally the Goom Gooruduron-yeran Campground is reached and soon after, the Coliban channel access track, after which it's a short stroll back to Blossett Drive.

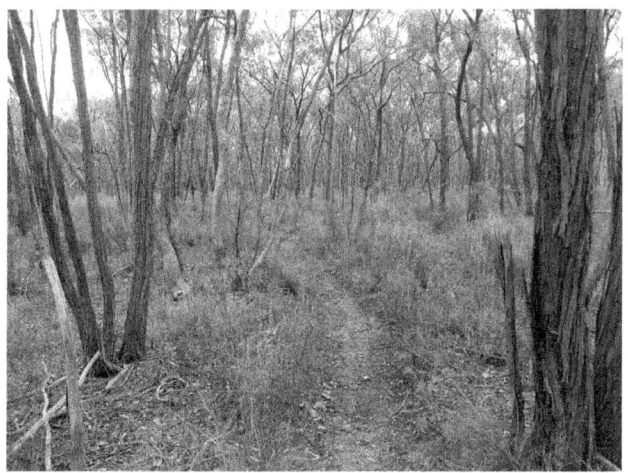

Return track to Blossett Drive.

You can tell when you've reached the edge of the Coliban water reserve by the ubiquitous concrete fence posts. Distinctive and everlasting, they must have made thousands of them.

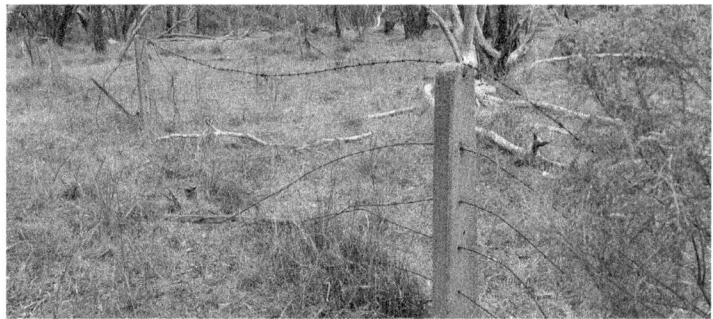

Harpers Road to Sandhurst Reservoir

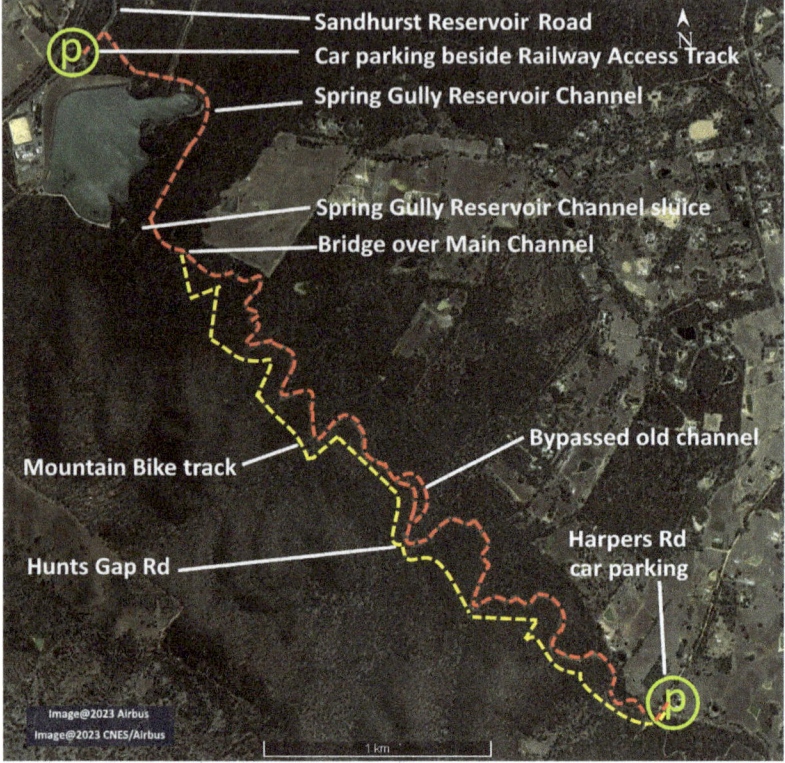

Again, walkers have a choice of a return walk of about 10 km or a car shuttle (one-way walk of 7.5 km). There is a car parking area at Harpers Road (see previous walk) and another just off Sandhurst Reservoir Road by the side of the railway access track near the Sandhurst Reservoir gates.

This section is similar to the previous walk, at least until Sandhurst Reservoir is reached. The environs of the channel are little different, as is the option of a return walk via the mountain bike trail winding its way through the Greater Bendigo National Park.

About one kilometre past Harpers Road, there is a large overshoot indicating the quantity of water which must from time to time pour from this upper catchment of Sheepwash Creek.

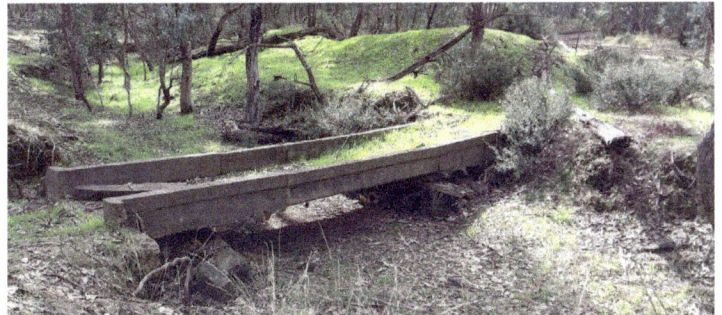

Overshoot on old channel near Harpers Road.

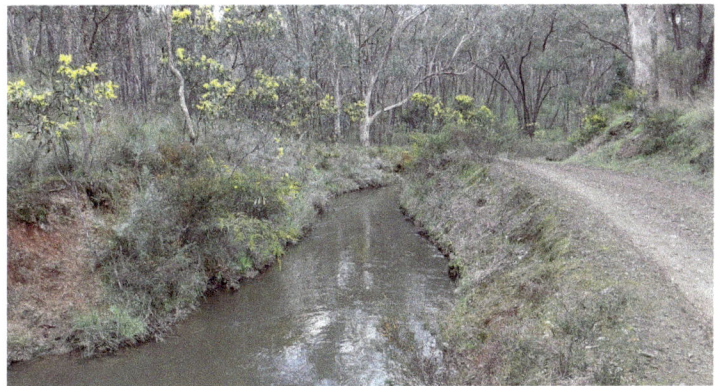

Channel and access road near Harpers Road.

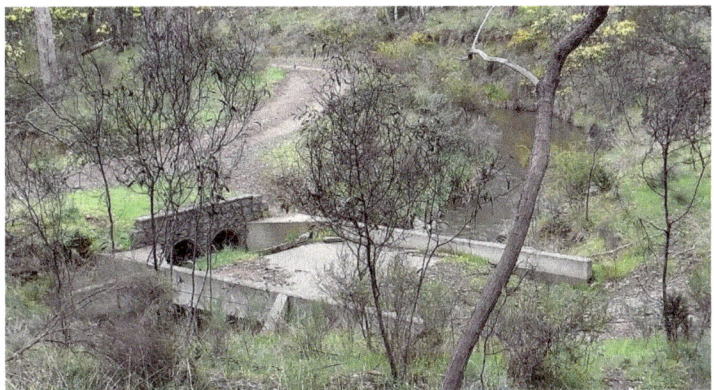

Large overshoot, Sheepwash Creek.

In about 800 metres, Hunts Gap Road crosses the channel. The old bridge and channel are worth a look, not least because a historic photo was taken at this location. It was here that an excited reporter in 1877 saw the signs of the initial flow from the Malmsbury Reservoir.

> 'We can now, however, authoritatively state that the water is running in a strong stream into the Big Hill [No. 7] Reservoir, and has been since Friday night. Our reporter inspected the channel on Saturday as far back as the crossing at Hunt's [Gap] road, where it was running along merrily about a foot deep, but rather muddy. He followed the channel to the sluice-gates of the branch channel to the Spring Gully Reservoir, and from thence to the crossing of the Melbourne road, where the water was tumbling down the drop at that point right royally, one mile from the Big Hill Reservoir, into which it is now running.'
> *Bendigo Advertiser, Monday 26 November 1877, p. 2.*

Just past Hunts Gap Road there is a vertical concrete pipe which, if you've walked all the way from Malmsbury Reservoir, reminds you of how tired you must feel (see photo page 164).

At this point the old channel passes under the access road and for a short distance runs along on the right-hand side of the track. This provides an opportunity to detour from the Leanganook track

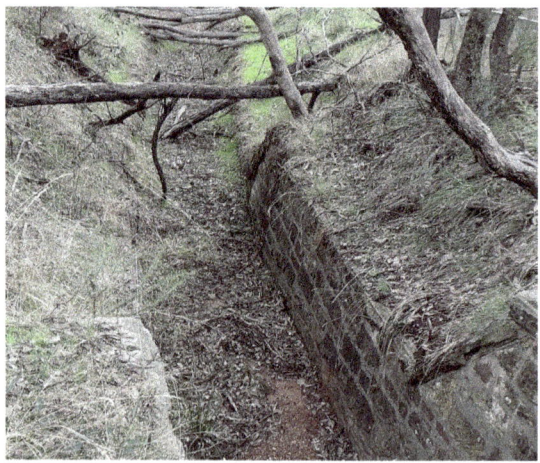

Old channel from Hunts Gap Road bridge looking north.

and follow the old channel. However, be warned, the foot track is somewhat indistinct and the going is a little rough. But it's always fun to walk along the old decommissioned channel, if only to get a sense of what it must have been like back in the nineteenth century. Almost immediately you will see another of the old brick sluice-gates.

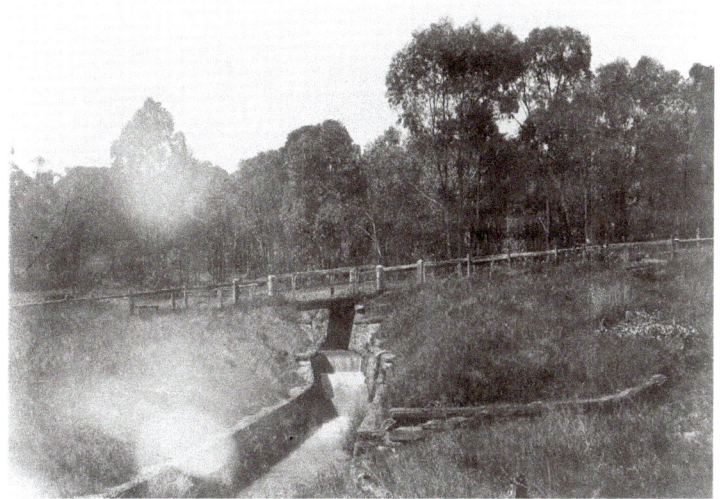
Hunts Gap Road, old channel, 1900.

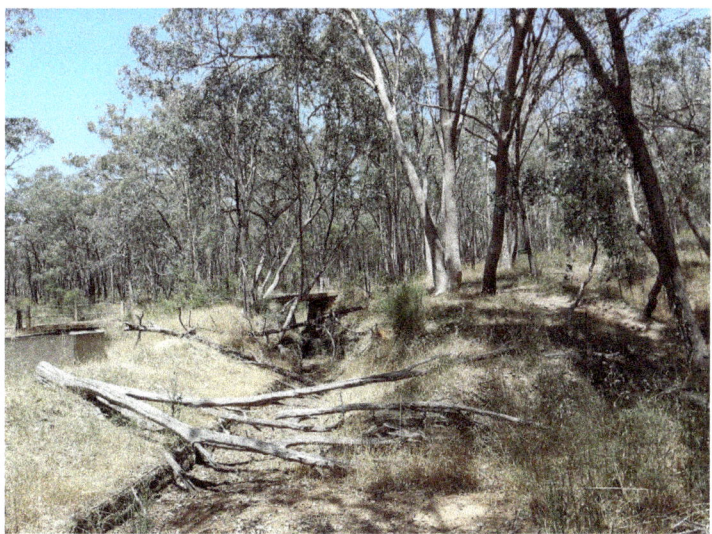
Present day view of old Hunts Gap Road bridge.

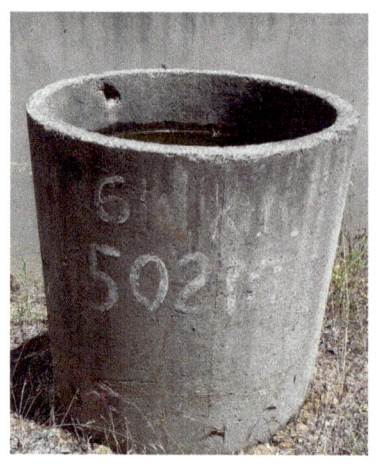

It's 61 km 502 m from Malmsbury Reservoir.

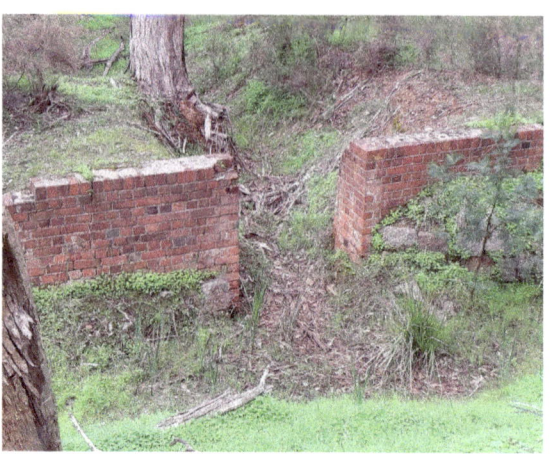

Sluice-gate, old channel east of Leanganook Track.

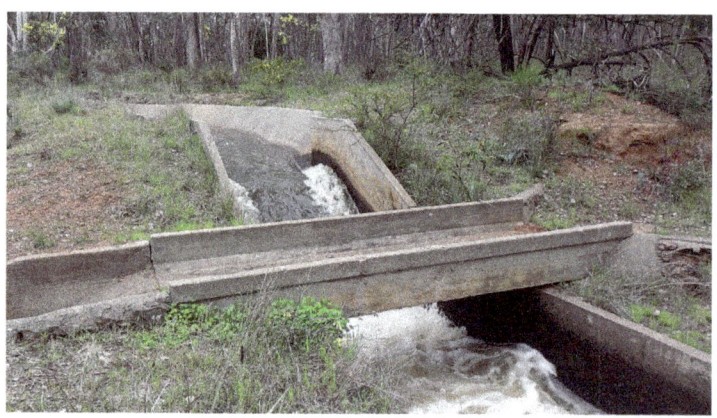

Drop (or gradient check) and overshoot, Mandurang.

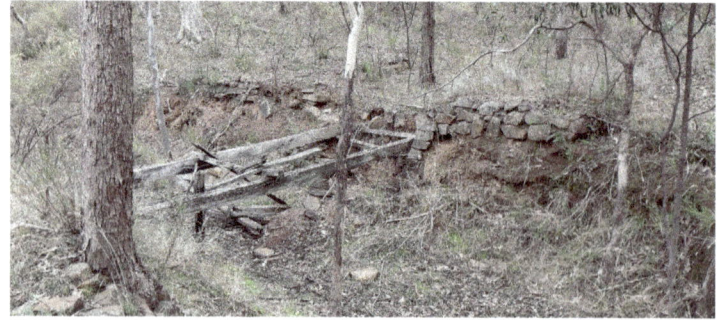

Remains of wooden overshoot, old Coliban channel.

It's not long before the old channel loops back to meet the current channel, just in time for a feature to pop into view, a drop in height and another overshoot.

In 900 metres, if you can find your way over to the old channel, you can see the ruins of one of a handful of remaining timber overshoots. They've long been replaced by overshoots made of concrete, so these must be very old, possibly from the 1920s or '30s. It proves there can't have been a destructive fire along this section of the channel for many years.

Further along, there is what seems to be a modern waste weir, designed to protect the channel when the water level becomes too high, perhaps during a major rain event. Whereas the original granite waste weirs (stormwater overpours) emptied the water on the lower (east) side, this weir empties the excess water on the west or uphill side. This has probably been done to protect the access track from damage. Run-off water is collected by a catchwater drain which channels the water back under a culvert into a gully on the east side.

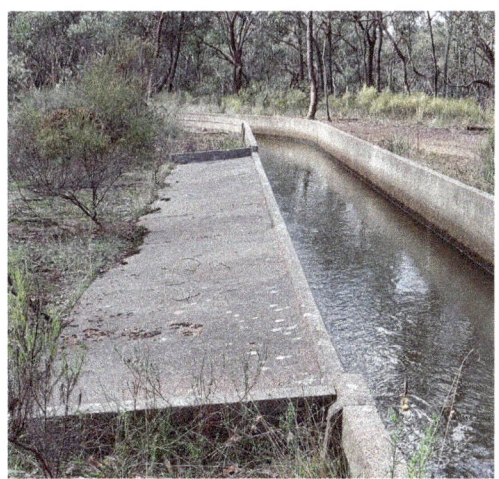

Flood overflow outlet.

Within 400 metres, the first of three metal bridges is met. Philip Wilkin[56] believes the two metal posts in the centre of these bridges are meant to deter dirt bikes. Not too successfully though, they're still managing to get over to that side by other means. However, it

---
56 Wilkin, p.74.

might prevent bikes and riders from suddenly finding themselves in the channel, these bridges are pretty slippery when wet.

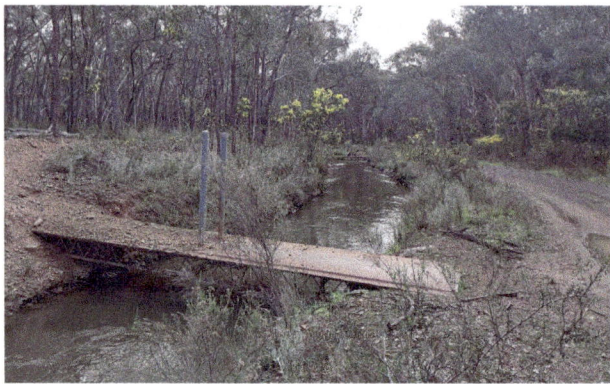

Metal bridge with dirt bike barrier.

At the 64 km mark[57] we come to a concrete overshoot and bridge. This one is less of a challenge for bike riders and kangaroos to cross. This is the recommended bridge across the channel for walkers returning to Harpers Road via the mountain bike path.

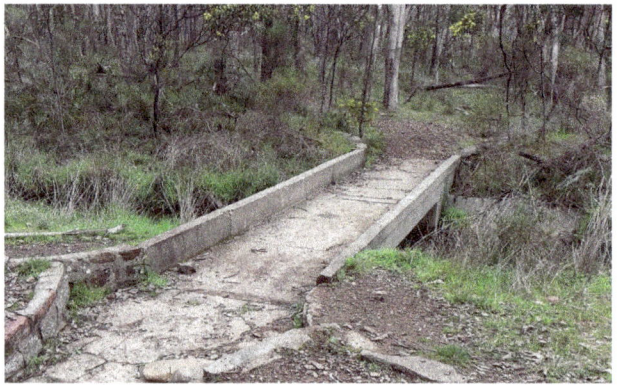

Concrete overshoot or bridge.

Hydraulic trash grates are a relatively recent addition to Coliban Water's infrastructure. They make the job of removing tree branches, dead animals and other rubbish a lot easier.

---

57 There is a metal distance marker fixed to the channel wall at this point.

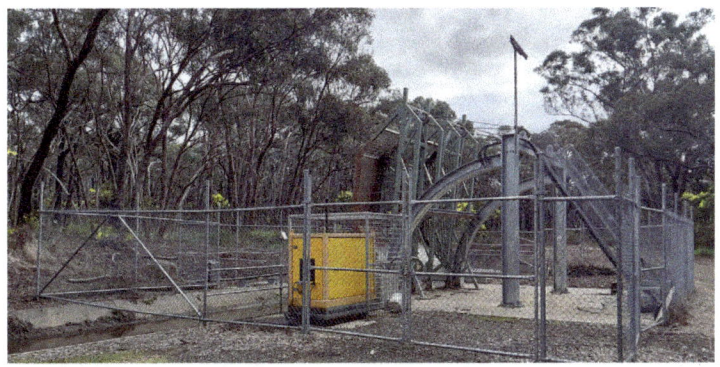
Trash grate, Sandhurst Reservoir.

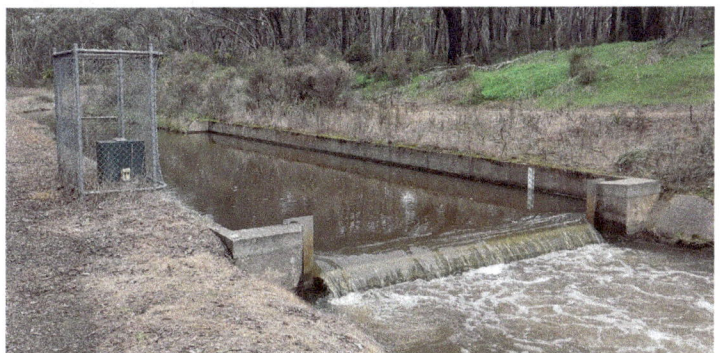
Weir, tank and measuring gauge.

About 100 metres or so past this there is a weir and tank with a measuring gauge.

And just ahead, finally, is Sandhurst Reservoir, one of the smaller reservoirs on the Coliban system. These days, Bendigo no longer relies so much on the water stored here. Lake Eppalock and the Waranga Basin provide the city with a major portion of its water needs.

Ahead, behind the chain link fence is the junction of the Main Channel and the Spring Gully Reservoir channel. The sluice-gates are somewhat altered but still retain some their original features.

> 'The Spring Gully junction is reached at 40¼ miles (64.8 km). Here, like at the beginning of the channel, sluices are erected, which can be opened or shut one or both at the same time.'
> Bendigo Advertiser, Tuesday 20 November 1877, p. 3.

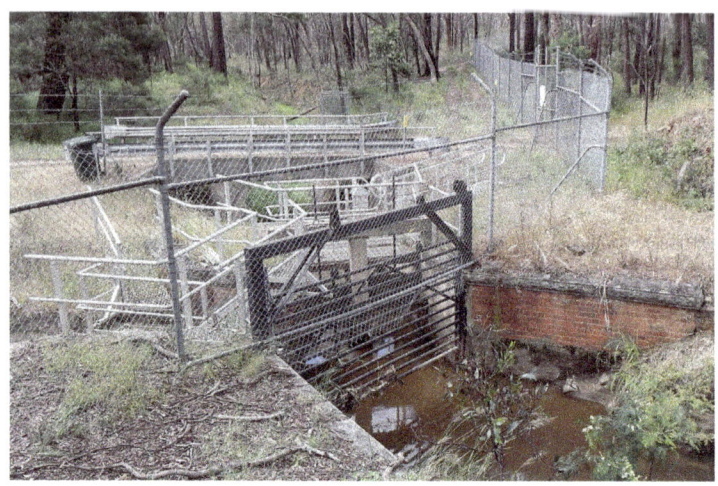
Spring Gully Channel sluice-gates.

Walkers now have a number of choices. Those who've arranged a car shuttle should head north along the Leanganook Track crossing over the Spring Gully Reservoir channel[58] where it emerges from behind the chain link fence, and then continue to follow the fence when it turns west. Shortly you will encounter a gravel road. Follow that to Sandhurst Reservoir Road, turn left and the car parking area is on your right just before the gates.

Walkers heading into Bendigo can either continue to follow the Leanganook Track which will lead you right into the heart of town to the Bendigo railway station. Alternatively, by following the railway track you can head to the Kangaroo Flat station.

If you decide to follow the Leanganook Track you will, for the first part at least, follow parallel to the Spring Gully Channel. A short detour to look at some of the features of this now decommissioned channel is worthwhile.

Those who wish to connect to the Three Reservoirs Circuit Walk (page 184) will follow the track that hugs the southern fenceline of the reservoir and then face another choice further

---

58 The Spring Gully Reservoir was originally intended to be a major dam supplying water to Sandhurst (as Bendigo was then called), but it proved unsatisfactory for a number of reasons: 'Its water is useless for domestic purposes unless it is filtered. That supplied by its own watershed is muddy, and when it was clarified by the admixture of water pumped out of the mines it became brackish.' *The Argus*, Saturday 7 August 1875, p. 4.

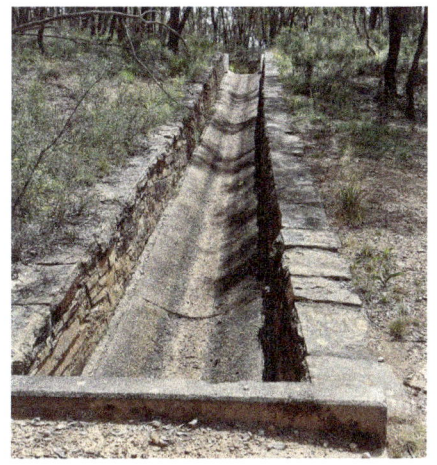 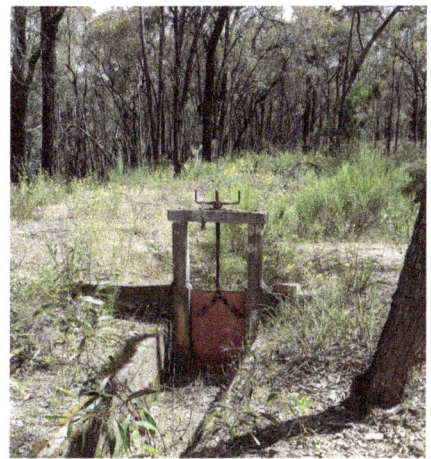

Features along Spring Gully Channel.

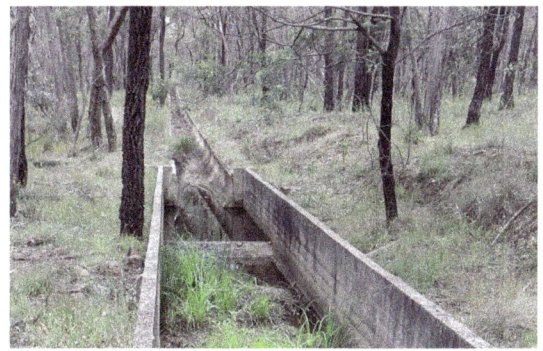

along – whether to follow the old main channel once it re-emerges from within the fenced Sandhurst Reservoir or follow the Big Hill High Level Reservoir channel after it too emerges from behind the chain link fence. Either way you're in for an adventure because neither walk is straightforward. Refer page 172 (Sandhurst Reservoir to No. 7 Reservoir).

But first, for those wishing to return to Harpers Road, here's a short description of the track through the Greater Bendigo National Park. Like the previous section, this alternative return route follows a mountain bike path which is also used by the occasional dirt bike. The path never ventures very far from the channel and so some of the previously unseen features of the original and now disused channel can be observed. I don't recommend crossing the channel via the very warped metal bridge near the start of the return walk (why only this bridge is so damaged is a puzzle). One of the bridges further back up the channel offers a safer option.

If you're walking through the Greater Bendigo National Park during spring you're sure to see a profusion of wildflowers. You'll also see a number of serious weeds, some of which are proving difficult to eradicate.

The track follows a fence line for a while. On the other side of the fence is a dam which has seen better days.

In no time at all you're back at Harpers Road and the car park.

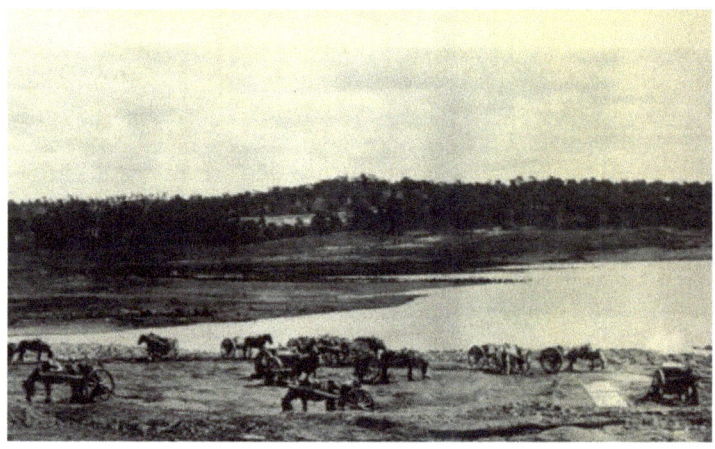

Spring Gully Reservoir 1927.

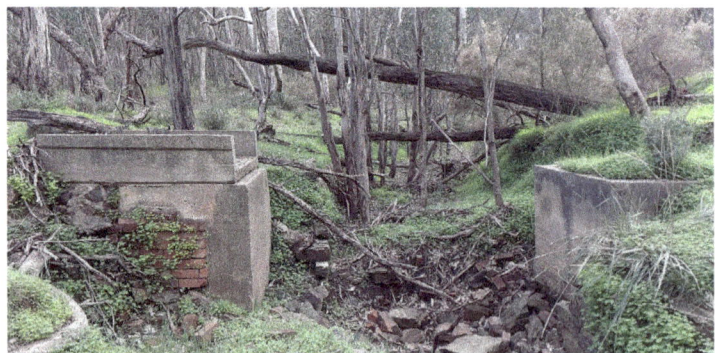

Ruins of concrete overshoot, old channel.

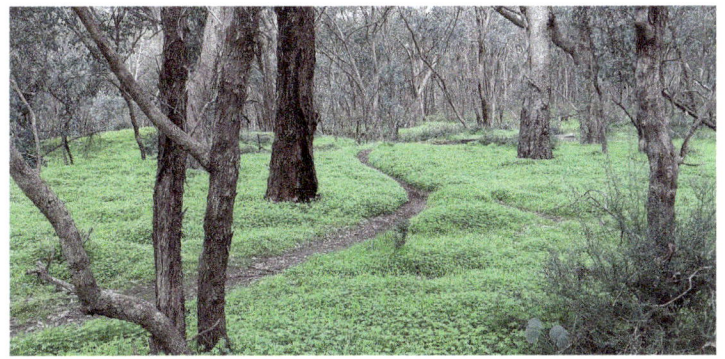

*A pretty green carpet? No, an infestation of Soursob (*Oxalis pes-caprae*).*

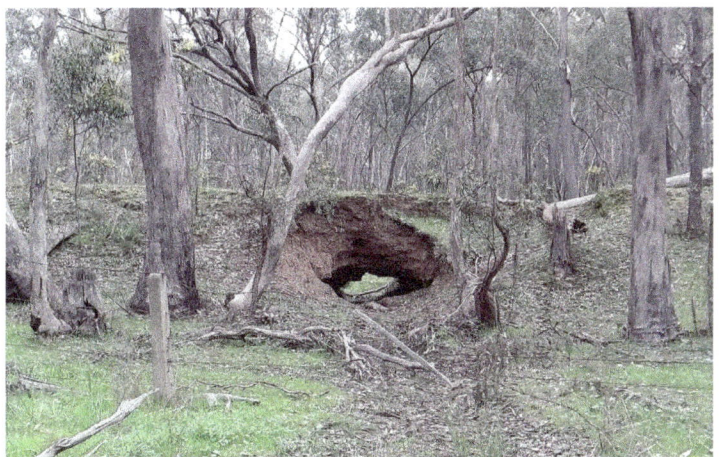

Washed out dam, mountain bike track.

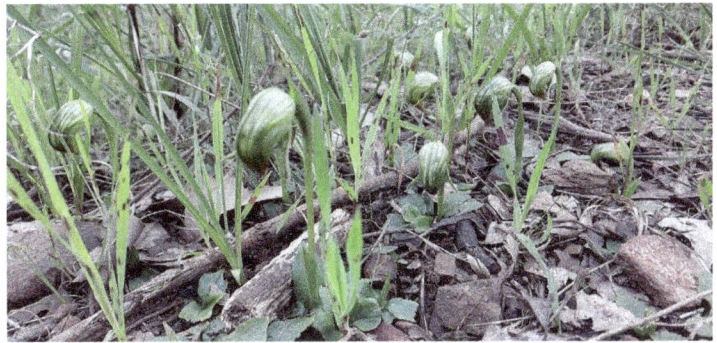

*Nodding greenhoods (*Pterostylis nutans*), definitely not a weed!*

Sandhurst Reservoir to No. 7 Reservoir

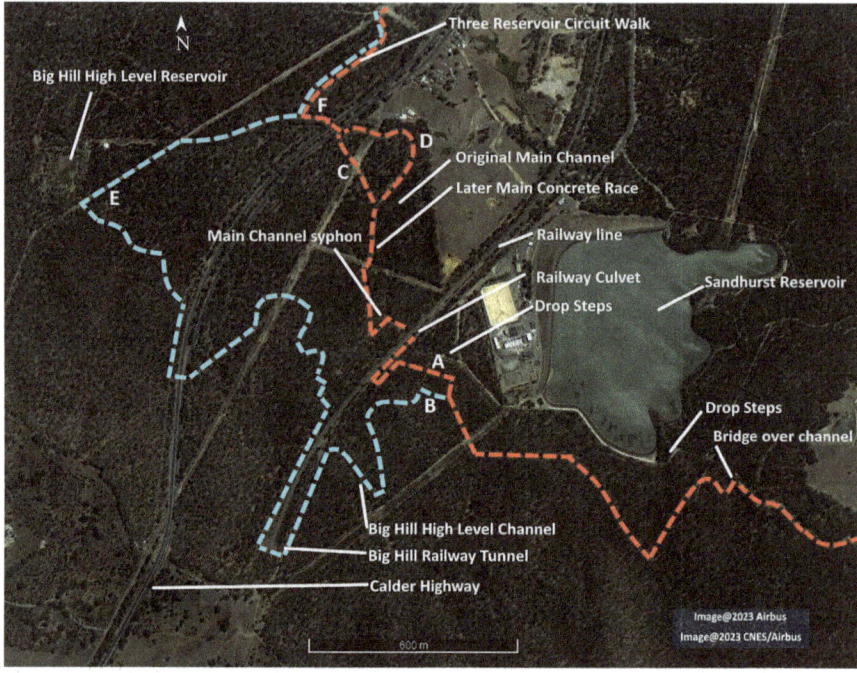

For those intrepid walkers intent on following the Main Channel from Sandhurst Reservoir to Crusoe Reservoir, the section between Sandhurst Reservoir and No.7 Reservoir is difficult going and not advisable for those simply seeking a pleasant diversion.

Because the Main Channel is now behind a chain link fence barrier, some of its historic features can't be viewed. And while there is a track along the fence perimeter, once over (or more accurately, under) the railway line there is no formal track along much of the channel. There is also the difficulty and danger of crossing a very busy Calder Highway. Walkers should carefully consider whether it's worth the effort and risk of exploring both the Coliban Main and Big Hill High Level channels in this area.

For those who wish to do so I'll now describe the two alternative routes (Main Channel path: A, High Level Channel path: B) from the end of the previous walk – the point where the channel enters Sandhurst Reservoir on the east side.

So, head over the bridge across the channel mentioned in the previous walk (page 166). Follow the chain link fence south-west. The fence will turn sharply north-west, and behind it, the channel drops through an interesting heritage stone structure composed of four steps. Above this, the Big Hill High Level Channel heads off to the south (to the right of this photo). It then follows a path of higher elevation to the now decommissioned Big Hill High Level Reservoir on the other side of the Calder Highway.

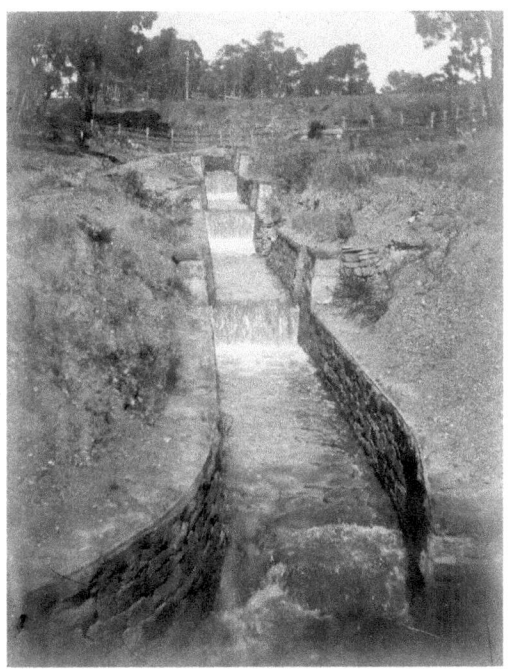

First lot of 4 steps, Sandhurst Reservoir, ca. 1900.

'From Spring Gully Junction there are two very fine Sluice gates across the main channel, and one across the Spring Gully race, which leaves the main channel, at an angle of about 60 degrees. Leaving the Spring Gully race, and following along the main channel, we come across a step drop about fourteen and a half feet deep ... This drop, unlike the others, is built with almost vertical walls at the sides. The bottom is formed into a flight of steps, like an ordinary staircase, only that the steps are much

larger and deeper. The reason for this design is that the full force and friction of the falling waters are broken and overcome at every step, and the wear and tear is no greater at the bottom than the top, but in other and simpler forms, the wear and tear is always much greater at the bottom than the top'.
The Age Thursday 3 January 1878 p. 3.

These days, most of the time, the water coming down the Main Channel is diverted into Sandhurst Reservoir, but when required by irrigators downstream, water still flows along the Channel to the Lockwood/Marong and Specimen Hill channels.

Continue along the perimeter fence. At one point the track turns into a narrow bike track and later crosses a pipeline easement and the Big Hill High Level channel. Here, you might choose to follow this channel. We'll return to this point later.

Near the railway line you will see another high chain link fence. But this appears to belong to VicTrack. This is a relatively recent addition. Quite why it's been erected is unclear as it doesn't stop anyone entering the reserve. It simply means one has to detour around and continue along the railway access track northwards through a gate which must be closed behind you.

Once through the gate, follow the access track until you come to a metal mesh bridge. The old main channel runs underneath this bridge.

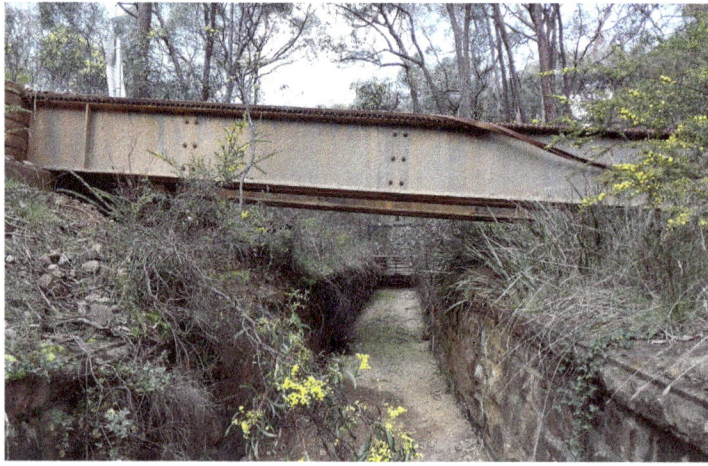

Metal mesh bridge over old main channel.

There is an old photo of the cascade of steps leading down to this point. Unfortunately, this series of ten steps is behind the fence, but we can glimpse part of it by peering through the chain links.

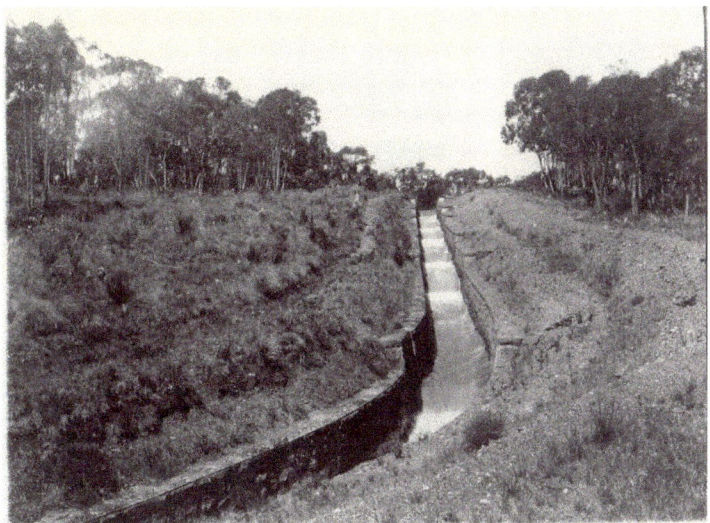

Second lot of steps near railway culvert.

'From this drop the channel meanders along the slopes of the hills to a point a few chains from the Mount Alexander railway at the ninety-fourth mile post from Melbourne, and about a quarter of a mile on the Sandhurst side of the Big-hill tunnel. Here another step drop like the last is met with. It is 1100 feet above the sea. The stream then runs under the railway and down a natural valley for about half a mile, where it again enters a race and follows the contour of the country until it reaches No. 7 or the Big Hill reservoir, which is 1000 feet above sea level. A good deal of work has been expended on this part of the channel on account of the bad nature of the ground for standing. Many of the banks have had to be protected by retaining walls'.
The Age, Thursday 3 January 1878 p. 3.

At least we don't have to cross the railway line. If the water isn't flowing down the old channel, we can walk under the railway line through the old culvert.

Once through the culvert you will be standing in an old stone-lined section of channel.

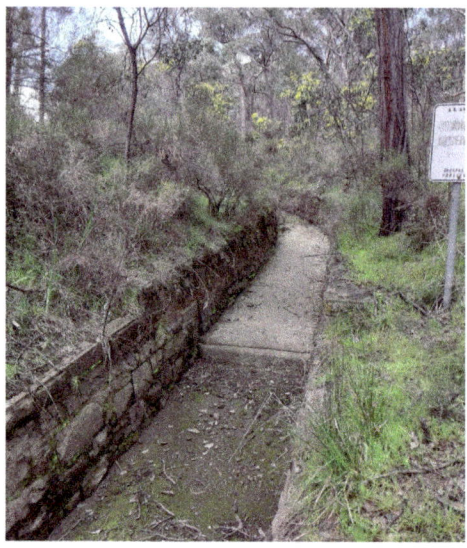

Old channel inside Sandhurst Reservoir reserve.

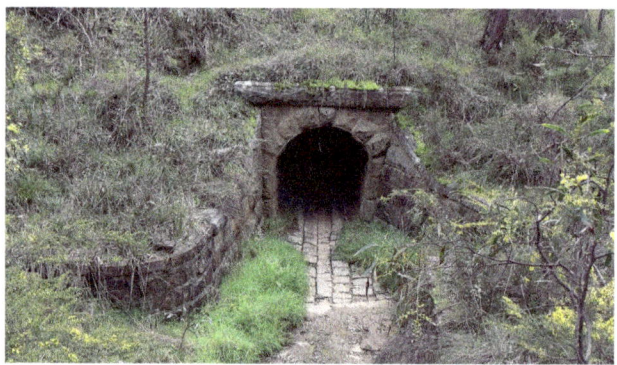

Culvert under the railway line.

'The channel crosses under the railway at 41 miles [66 kms], when it follows a natural watercourse, which has been formed by masonry into a drop, consisting of a series of steps, passing under the railway through a masonry culvert, 7 feet by 4 feet, very strongly and handsomely built, with circular arch and invert, all of granite.'
Bendigo Advertiser, Tuesday 20 November 1877, p. 3.

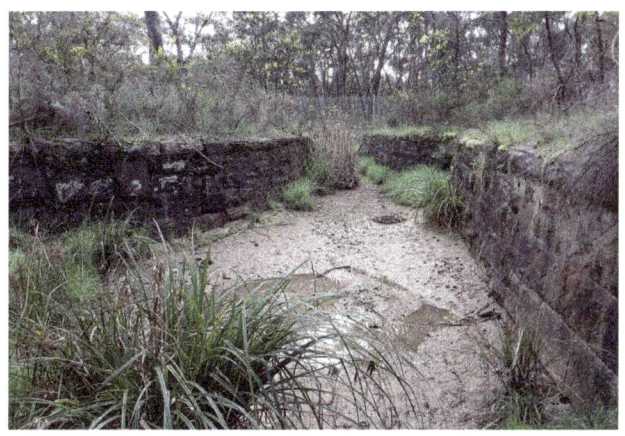

Main channel between railway culvert and Calder Highway.

Originally, the channel took advantage of a natural watercourse to funnel the waters down to the Melbourne Road (Calder Highway). But this meant, just as it did on the Expedition Pass Reservoir channel, weirs and steps had to be constructed to prevent the scouring of the banks. This must have proved unsuccessful because at some stage it was decided to bypass the creek and build a new channel to the west. A syphon was installed to transport the water under the creek to the new water race.

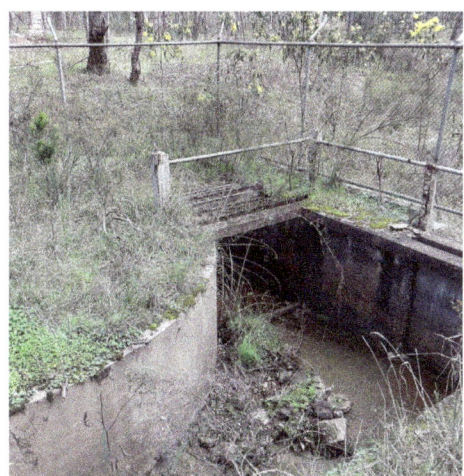

Later syphon on left, sluice to old channel on right.

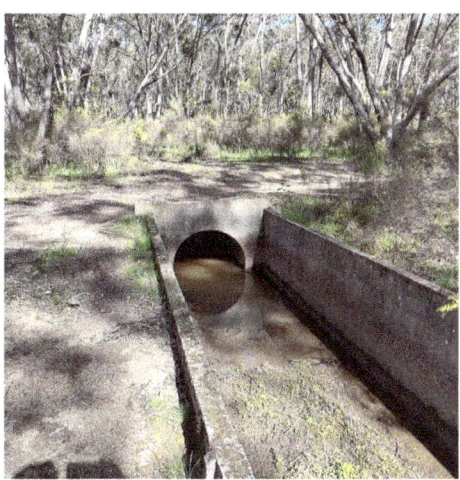

Main channel syphon outlet.

A track heads off west here. It leads to the syphon outlet near the next track junction.

In about 300 metres the track heads away from the channel to the left. The easiest and recommended path is to continue along this track to the Calder Highway (C). Others might prefer to continue along the indistinct path that follows the channel (D). (See map page 172.)

At the end of a steep narrow chute[59] the original channel which had utilised the natural watercourse joins the water race.

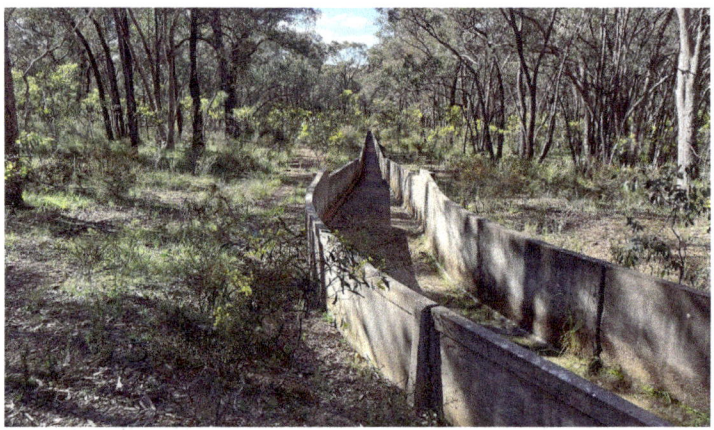

Water race between the railway line and Calder Highway.

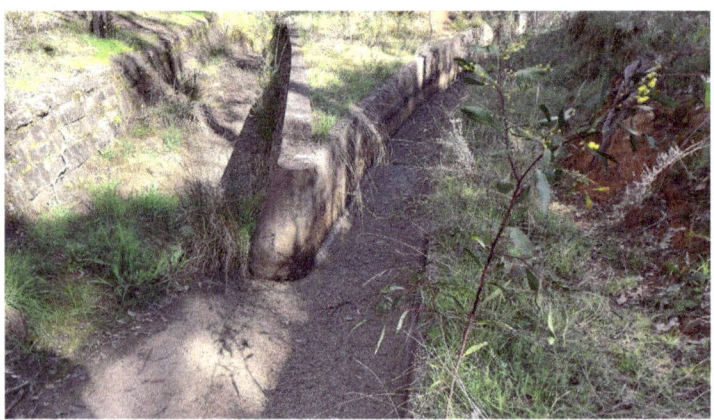

Original channel on left, later water race on right.

---

59 The steeper the channel, the narrower it can be to facilitate the same flow.

'From this, the drop continues all along the natural watercourse to near the Melbourne road. The aggregate fall of these steps cannot be under 60 [18.3 m] or 70 feet.'
Bendigo Advertiser, Tuesday 20 November 1877, p. 3.

From this point on you will follow one of the oldest original sections of the Main Channel. As the path grows increasingly indistinct it might be tempting to walk along the floor of the channel. However, given the uncertainty surrounding incoming flows I'd advise against it.

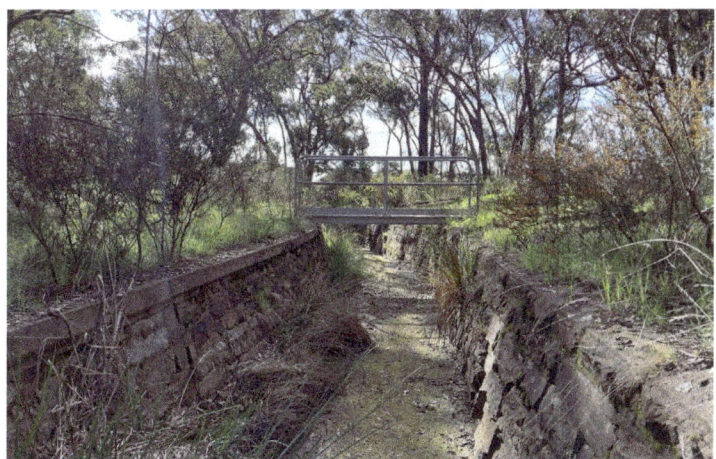

Footbridge over the old channel.

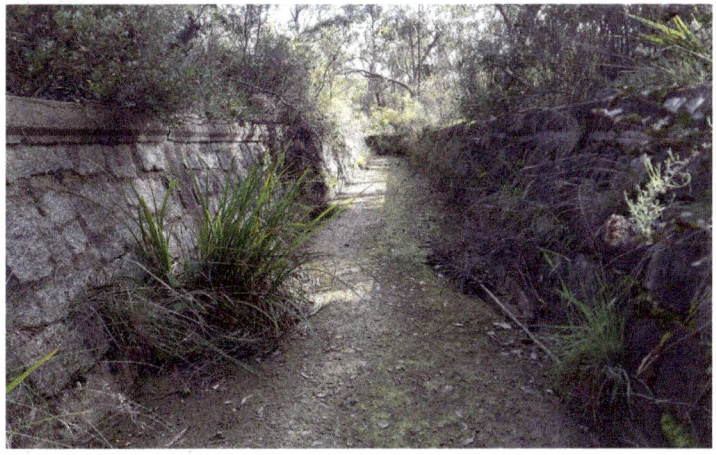

Approaching the Calder Highway culvert.

Unfortunately, the culvert under the Calder Highway is too low for pedestrians. There's no other option but to take one's chances and cross the highway. Luckily, it's a divided carriageway with a wide median strip to give you ample time to catch your breath.

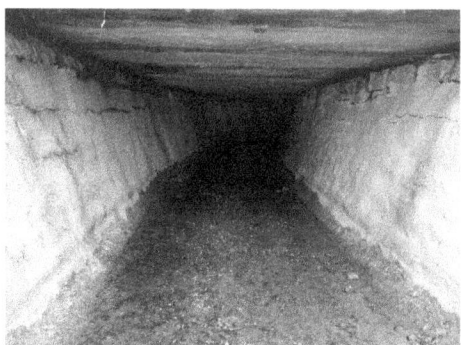

Culvert under Calder Highway.

The Main Channel to the west of the Calder Highway will be dealt with in the next section, The Three Reservoirs Circuit Walk. Walkers crossing the Calder will be following the last part of this walk (F) and should refer to the track notes on page 200.

An alternative to following the old Main Channel across to the west side of the Calder Highway is to head off along the Big Hill High Level channel (see map page 172, blue dashed line: B). However, this is even more challenging than following the Main Channel to the west of the highway. Again, this is probably the preserve of the inveterate field rambler, there being no discernible path along the High Level channel.

But for those willing to accept the challenge, soon after heading off along the High Level channel you will find another ruined wooden overshoot.

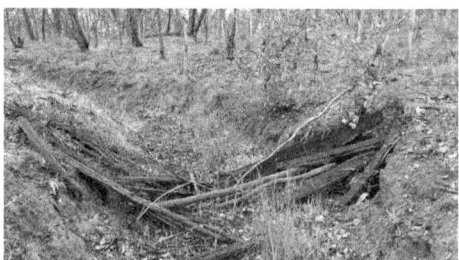

Remains of a wooden overshoot.

The plants growing in the channel here may look rather pretty but bulbil watsonia is a proclaimed noxious weed in Victoria. It's a scourge along many parts of the Main Channel as well as along drainage lines in a number of the nature reserves in this region.

The Bendigo rail line is just ahead. Unfortunately, there's no railway culvert to use as an underpass here. You may choose to cross the railway line, but the safe option is to make a detour and cross above the Big Hill railway tunnel, 300 metres to the south. It's worth having a closer look at this feature anyway.

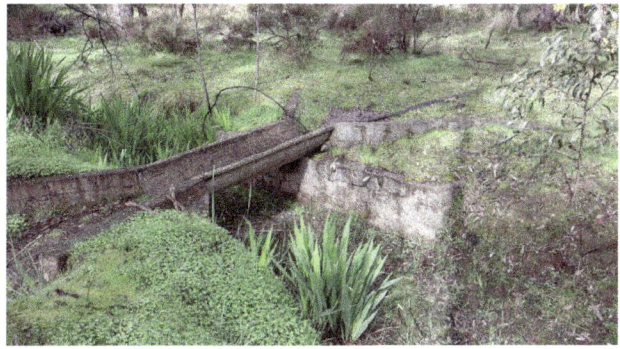

Concrete overshoot on Big Hill High Level Channel.

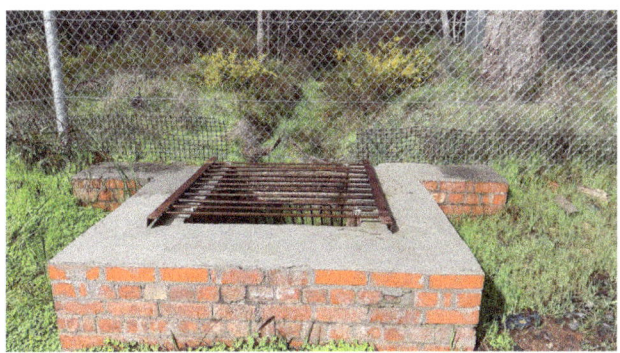

Syphon under railway line.

At the time of its construction in 1856, the Bendigo line was the largest engineering project in the Colony of Victoria. The 390 metres long tunnel at Big Hill is the longer of the two tunnels on the line. The other is at Elphinstone, not far from the Poverty Creek channel syphon which once carried water from Malmsbury Reservoir under the railway line.

Within 300 metres the channel crosses an unnamed track.

The channel crosses the Calder Highway via a nondescript culvert. At this point the highway is divided by a generous median strip which makes the crossing of the road a little less anxiety inducing.

Across the highway there is a track of sorts which leads to the continuation of the High Level channel. This path then accompanies the channel all the way to Lookout Track which links with the Three Reservoirs Walk (E). (See the next walk).

There are some pretty little bridges on this final section of the High Level channel.

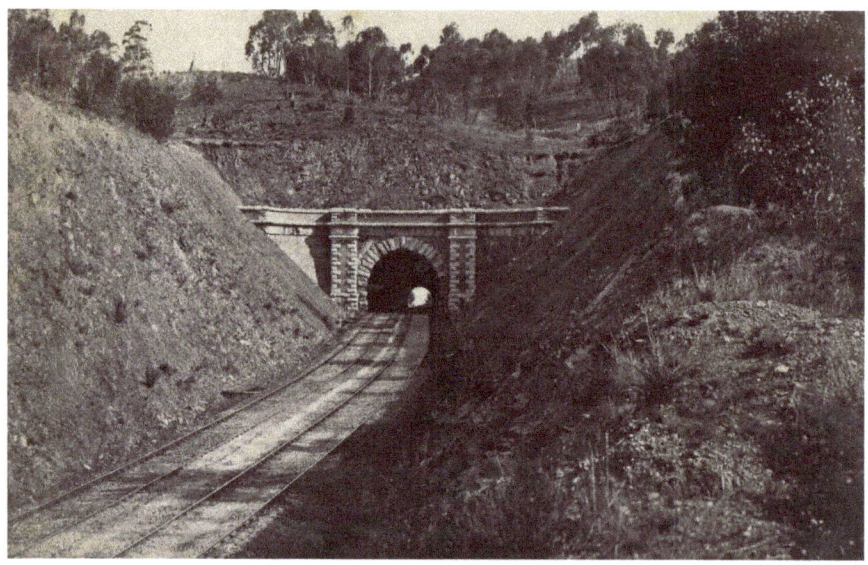

Southern entrance, Big Hill railway tunnel.

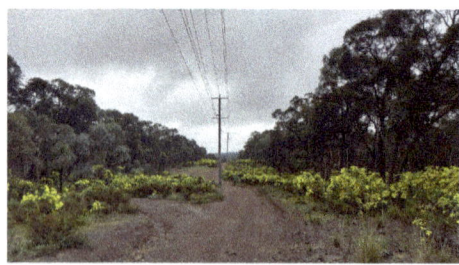

Power line easement track.

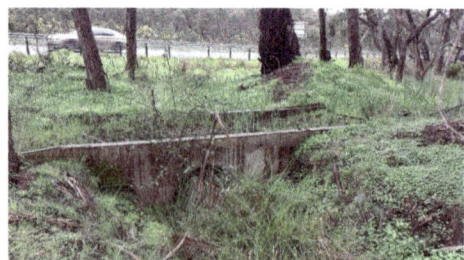

Culvert inlet, Calder Highway, Big Hill.

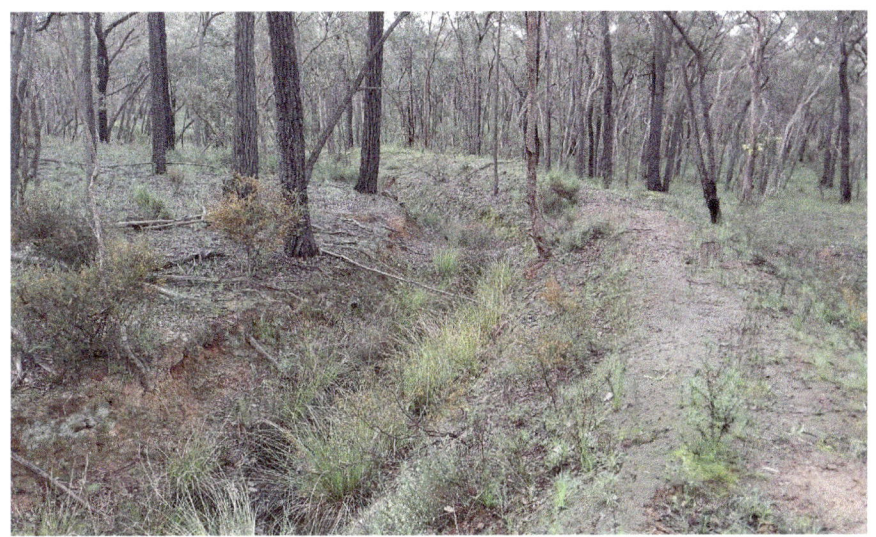

Big Hill High Level Channel west of Calder Highway.

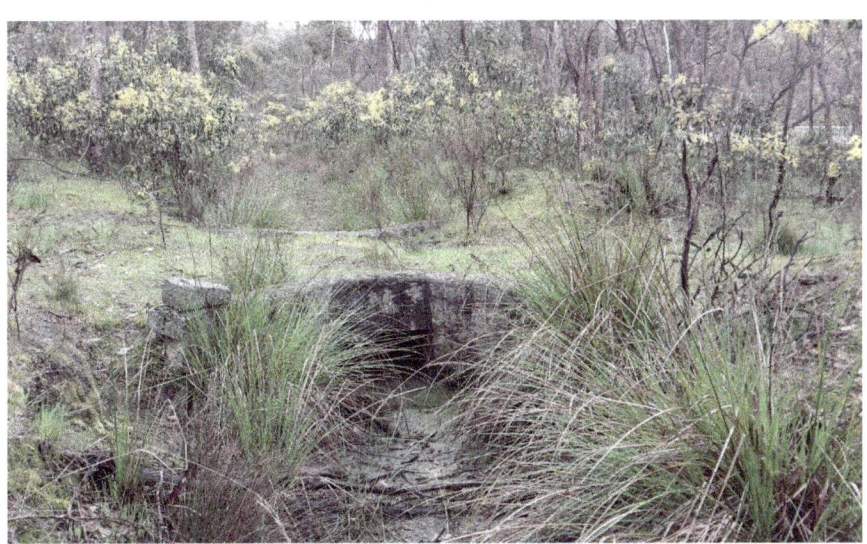

Bridge near Lookout Track, High Level Channel.

The Three Reservoirs Circuit Walk

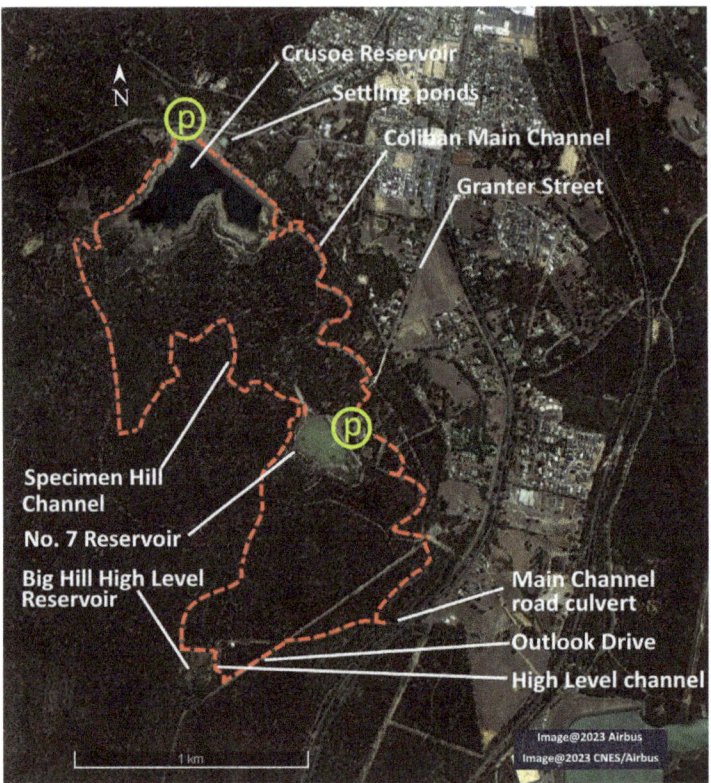

The starting point for this rewarding return walk of about 11 kilometres can either be the No. 7 Reservoir car park or the Crusoe Reservoir car park. Those who have crossed the highway by following the previous walk will, if following the Main Channel, join the circuit either at a pipeline easement track on the west side of the Calder Highway, or if following the High Level channel, at Outlook Track near the Big Hill High Level Reservoir (see map page 172).

Because the main aim of this book is to describe the Main Channel from Malmsbury Reservoir to Crusoe Reservoir, we will walk in an anticlockwise direction starting at the No. 7 Reservoir car park.

The No. 7 Reservoir can be reached via Granter Street (off Furness St), Kangaroo Flat, Bendigo. There are gardens, toilets and

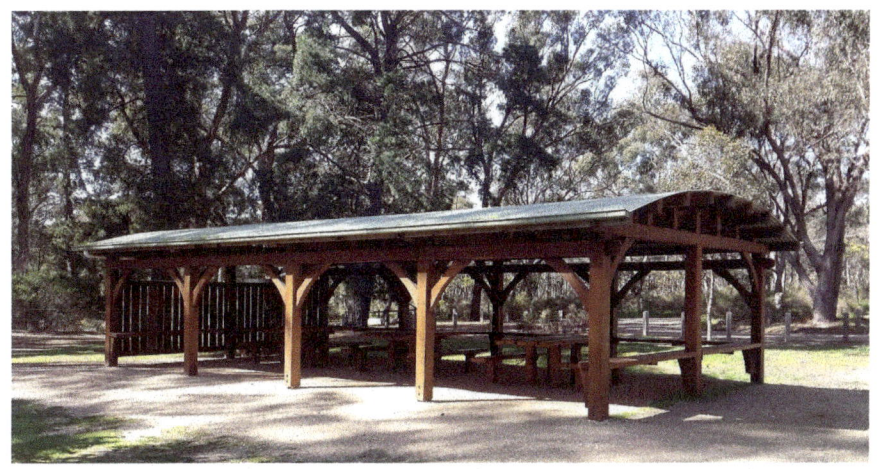

Shelter, No. 7 Reservoir, Granter Street, Big Hill.

a shelter, as well as many historical relics. This reservoir was one of the first constructed in Bendigo and was one of a series planned for Bendigo.

This walk takes in the three reservoirs in this area and offers a chance to walk some way along four channels or races. The gardens and surroundings are well worth an inspection before setting out, or on completion of the walk.

As already discussed, the engineer Joseph Brady was a central character in the early development of Victoria. His talents seemed to be at the centre of a large number of important projects. In 1863 he had put forward a scheme for supplying Bendigo and Castlemaine with water harvested from the Upper Coliban River catchment and impounded at a new reservoir to be built at Malmsbury. Within a few years his plan was accepted, and one of the first reservoirs built, as part of his ambitious scheme, was the No. 7 Reservoir (then also known as the Big Hill Reservoir).[60] He had planned the construction of eight reservoirs, most reserved for mining purposes due to the demand for water by mining companies. This pressure was irresistible owing to the immense wealth being generated by the extraction of gold. Sandhurst Reservoir is approximately where Brady's No. 8 reservoir would have been located.

---

60 The name Big Hill Reservoir for No.7 Reservoir appeared to fall out of favour when the Big Hill High Level Reservoir was constructed in 1882, presumably to avoid confusion.

The construction of No.7 Reservoir began on 27 May, 1859, and finished in June, 1860.

> 'About 40 men are employed in the completion of this work, which presents but little difficulty, owing to the judicious selection of the site. The only excavation rendered necessary is just a sufficiency of material for the formation of the embankment, which extends a distance of 320 yards across from the hill, which on three sides form a natural basin for the reception of the storm water from the adjacent ranges. This reservoir is of considerable extent, and the greatest depth will be about 30 feet. ... altogether the works evince an amount of skill highly creditable to the projectors of the undertaking'.
> *Bendigo Advertiser, Monday 28 November 1859, p. 3.*

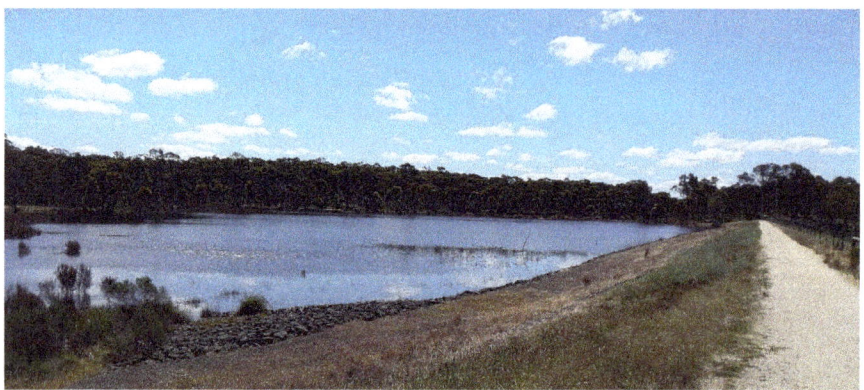

No. 7 Reservoir.

> 'The beautiful lake-like expanse of water [at No. 7 Reservoir] is naturally suggestive of a bath, and we hinted as much, but our obliging mentor, Mr A. A. Broadfoot, the resident superintendent of the works, quickly dispelled any idea of indulging in such a luxury by informing us that a fine of £5 awaited any rash person caught bathing there'.
> *The Star, Friday 15 November 1861, p. 3.*

Beginning at the car park, walk through the gardens to the path which passes between two stately pine trees. Behind the fence on the left are the remnants of the treatment works, settling beds and an enormous underground cistern, storage for the treated water.

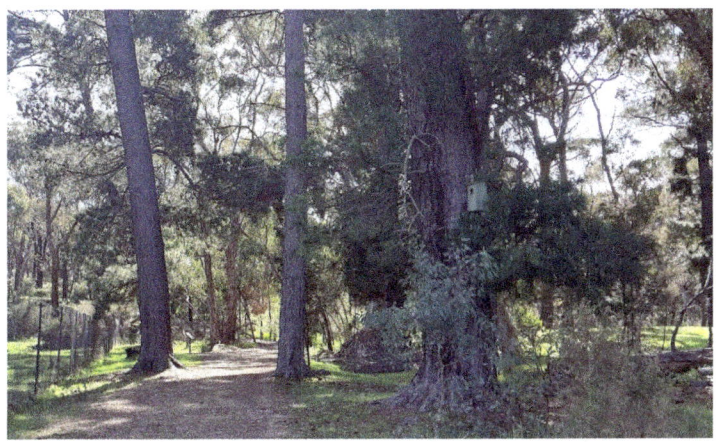
Start of the Three Reservoirs Circuit, No. 7 Reservoir.

'Below the dam bank are the gravitation and nitration beds or chambers, which we may describe as two large sunken chambers in brick work 45 feet square, by a depth of eleven feet. …. The clean water culvert then goes on to the receiving chamber, fifty feet in length by twenty five feet in width, with a depth of sixteen feet; the bottom and sides being built and puddled as in the filtration beds. In this are twelve brick pillars, on which will spring a series of arches, the whole will then be covered in with earth, and soiled over, to ensure coolness. From this there is a valve to the main leading down to Sandhurst'.
The Star, Friday 15 November 1861, p. 3.

This underground cistern, long fallen into disuse, had been lost to memory. It was rediscovered in 1964 when a backhoe broke through the roof of the structure. Apparently, as early as 1903, the treatment works had been abandoned.

' Close at hand are some settling beds, but they are too small to be of use nowadays, having been constructed at a time when the consumers of water were few. The beds have not been used for many years'.
Bendigo Advertiser, Thursday 19 February 1903, p. 2.

Take the right-hand fork at the next track junction. Alongside this path is the No. 7 Park Frog Ponds – a re-creation of what the Bendigo Creek might have once looked like. About 200 metres on, the road is met. The old Main Channel is on the other side of the road behind a fence and is inaccessible. Follow the path next to the road and cross the footbridge ahead.

Although there are paths on either side of the channel it's best to follow the northern path as it hugs the channel almost all the

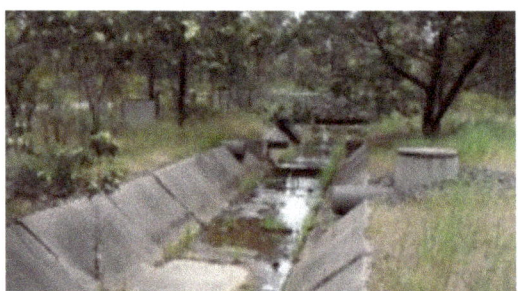

Channel at No. 7 Reservoir.

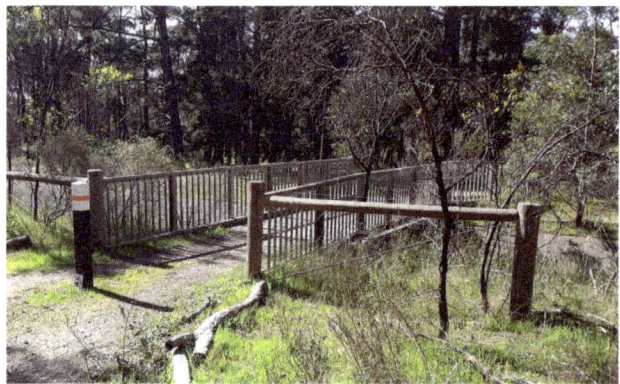

Footbridge over the Main Channel.

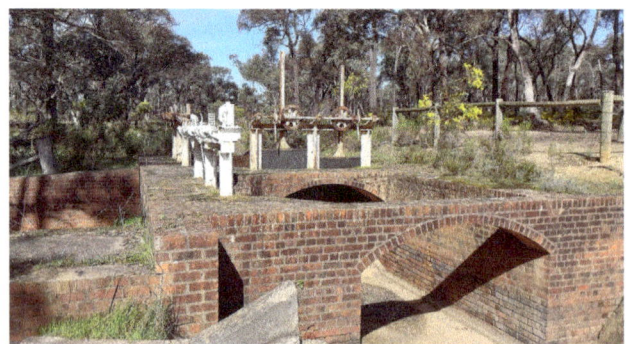

Sluice-gates, Crusoe Reservoir.

way to Crusoe Reservoir. At the end of the path are historic sluice-gates which once regulated the flow of water into Crusoe Reservoir.

> 'About 10 chains from the reservoir three sets of iron flood-gates are erected, known as the south sluices. One set to stop the passage of water down the channel into the reservoir,

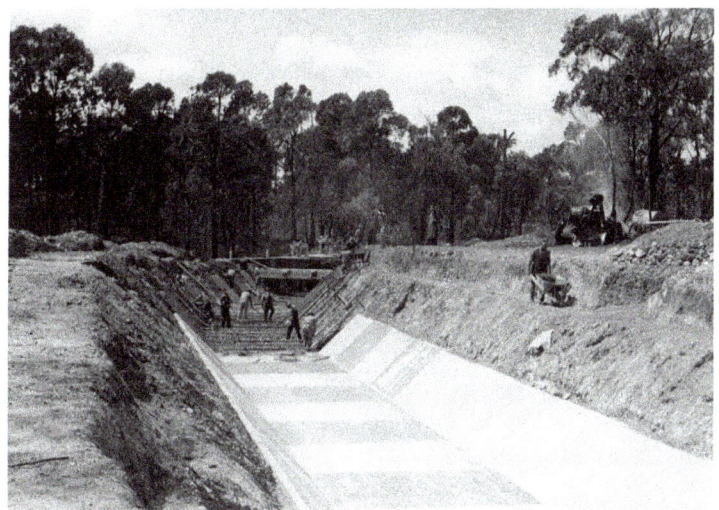

Main Channel near Crusoe Reservoir, sluice-gates in background, 1940, SR&WSC. Below: Present day view.

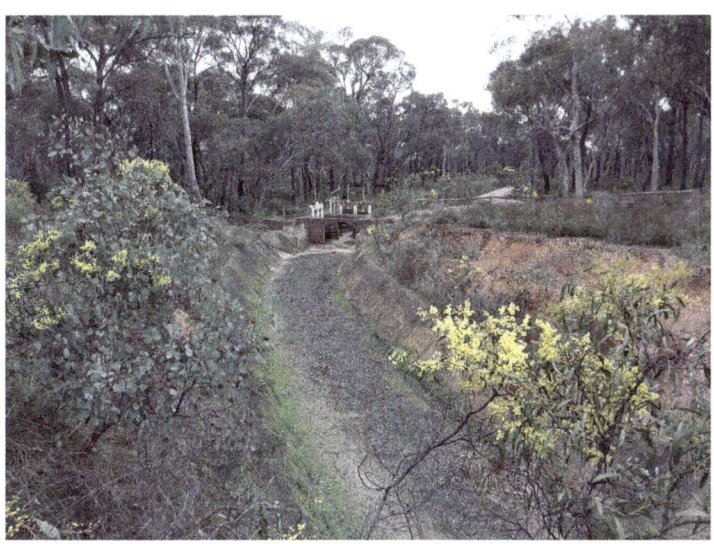

and one lateral set to convey the water so stopped into one of the side gullies away from the dam. The bye-washes are so arranged as to deliver floodwaters quite clear of the settling-ponds reserve, so that these may be guarded against all damage from flood. The third set of flood gates is also fixed in the side of the aqueduct, but on the reservoir side of the stop-gates, and the sill is fixed at 939 feet above sea-level so as to relieve the main bye-wash in case of an extreme flood'.
Bendigo Advertiser, Thursday 12 February 1874, p. 2.

Turn left almost immediately and cross the bridge. Then turn right to head towards the reservoir. A glimpse of Crusoe Reservoir can be seen through the trees, and shortly, if you turn right at the next path you will be able to see the last few metres of the channel, now resembling a natural stream bed leading into the reservoir.

Continue across the small bridge over the channel and soon you will come to the embankment. It looks like a long walk to the other end, and it is!

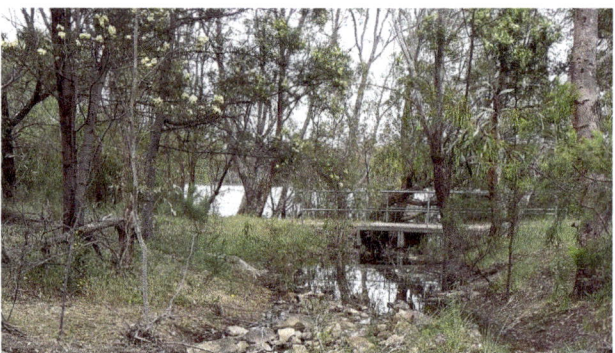

The last few metres of the old Coliban Main Channel.

'As soon as the City Council secured possession of the property of the Bendigo Waterworks, they took steps to raise funds to ... get a sufficient supply of water for the present increasing requirements of the city and the district ... They next appointed Mr. Brady, formerly engineer to the Bendigo Waterworks Company, to report, respecting the advisability of the best course to pursue. In the first instance it was proposed to

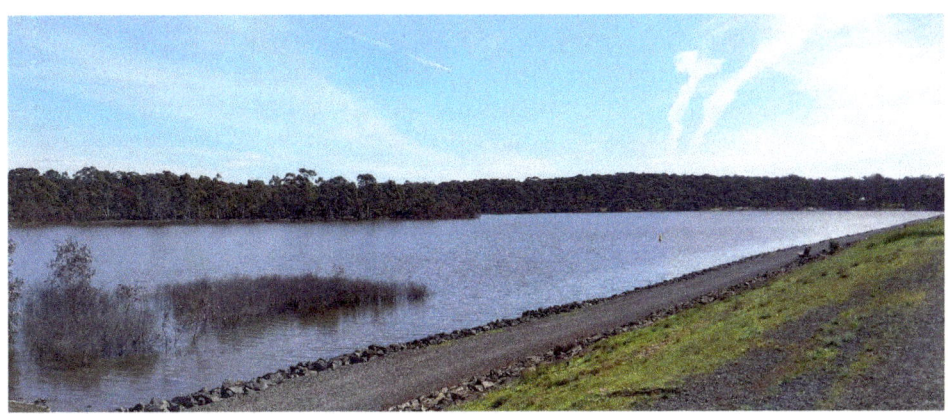

Crusoe Reservoir.

> construct a reservoir in the Anderson's Flat Valley,[61] which was originally a part of the Coliban scheme, but being recommended by Mr. Brady to construct a new reservoir in Robinson Crusoe Gully, the Anderson's Flat scheme was abandoned, and ever since, the efforts of the council have been directed to secure the latter object. Mr. Brady considers that the Crusoe site is a magnificent one, and has advantages far superior to any supplied by Anderson's Flat.'
>
> Bendigo Advertiser, 23 May 1872, p. 2.

Now you come to the embankment. If you walk along the top of the embankment you can see the original treatment plant on your right.

> 'Sandhurst also draws supplies from two other reservoirs, but Crusoe is the largest. This basin was originally a low-lying piece of ground, through which a watercourse, known as Robinson Crusoe Gully, ran, and hence the present name. ... The most interesting features about this work are the settling ponds. These are three in number, each about 50 yards square, and of brick construction faced with cement. There is no tower at Crusoe; but the water is sent to the ponds through a pipe, the receiving end of which is bent, to take the water above the silt bed. Thence it passes into the settling ponds. In the two first ponds the water is treated with lime, and then let into a third

---

61 According to an 1867 map of the proposed scheme this reservoir would have been close to the location of the current Big Hill High Level Reservoir.

basin, whence it goes to the Sandhurst main. The lime effects a wonderful change in the way of clarification ; for, though the water is quite yellow before reaching the lime ponds, it is clear and sparkling after entering the third basin. It naturally tastes strong of the lime, though this is a wholesome quality (only too often lacking in Australian water), but its passage through the Sandhurst pipes seems to remove all disagreeable taste; for, when drawn from a city tap it is certainly superior to a glass of the Yan Yean.'
The Sydney Morning Herald, Monday 1 February 1886 p. 6.

'Some time ago no little stir was made respecting the alleged pollution of the bed of the Crusoe reservoir through its having at one time received the drainage from a slaughter-yard, and

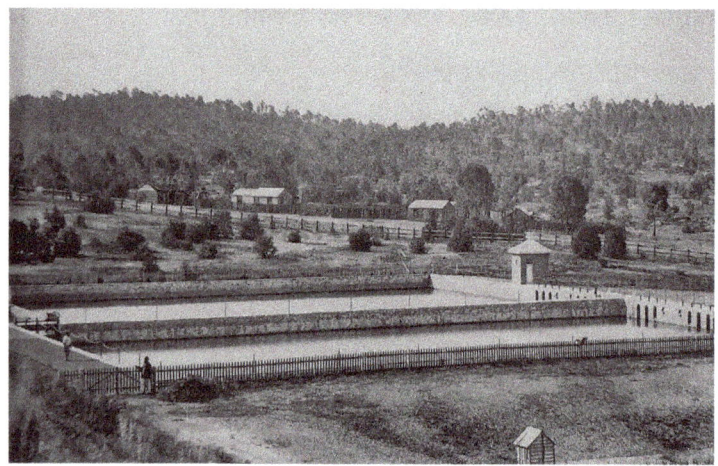

Settling ponds Crusoe Reservoir ca 1875. Below: As they are today.

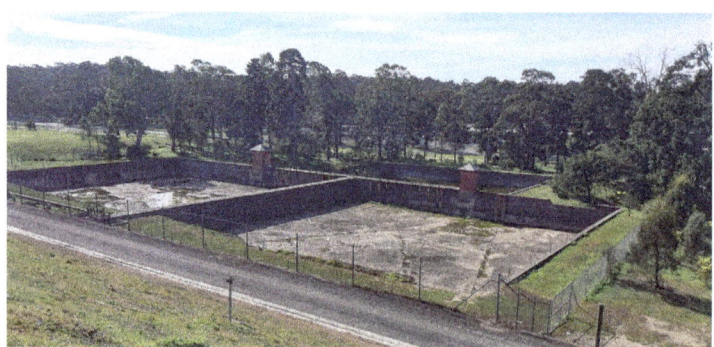

being within the immediate drainage area of a few houses. It was also stated that directly in the course of the natural channel which runs through the gully, an immense quantity of bones and other refuse from the abattoirs alluded to had been buried ... There is also a legendary Chinese camp buried deep beneath the waters that at present fill the lower portion of the reservoir; but the most critical examination of the spot itself, and of the traditions of the place, fail to give any clue to the history of this Australian Fair city, 'neath translucent waters buried'.
Bendigo Advertiser, Thursday 12 February 1874 p. 2.

As both No. 7 and Crusoe Reservoir are decommissioned they are available for recreation purposes. On any day people can be seen enjoying themselves walking, bike riding or fishing.

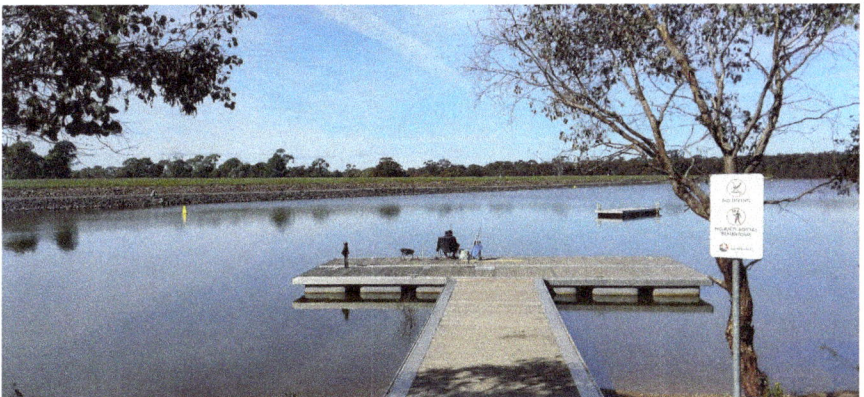

When you reach the end of the embankment, turn left to follow the lakeside track. In about 800 metres you will reach a crossroads. Turn right, away from the reservoir, and then turn left at the next junction. This track appears to be unnamed. In about 500 metres you will cross (Robinson) Crusoe Gully, a name which pre-dated the building of the reservoir. In another 400 metres you will come to the Specimen Hill channel and another track junction.

> 'The party then proceeded to inspect portions of the route of the proposed Specimen Hill aqueduct. It is intended to carry the aqueduct from a point above the Big Hill Reservoir along the summit of the range on the northern side of the Bendigo Creek

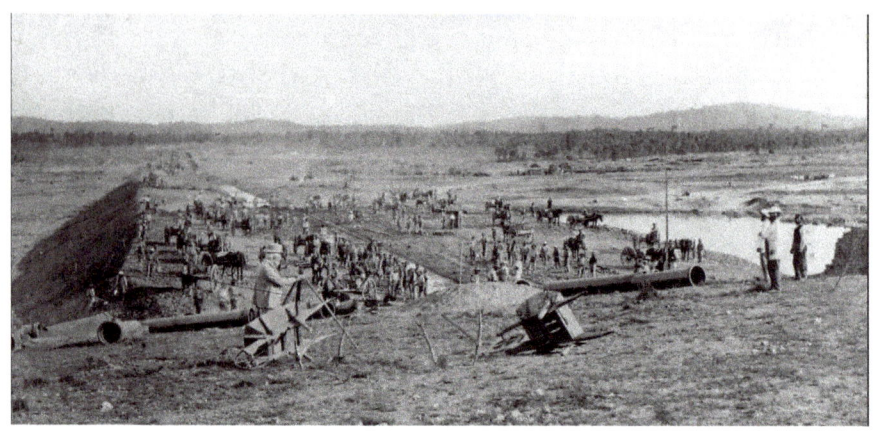

Crusoe Gully Reservoir during construction, 1872. Below: Present day view.

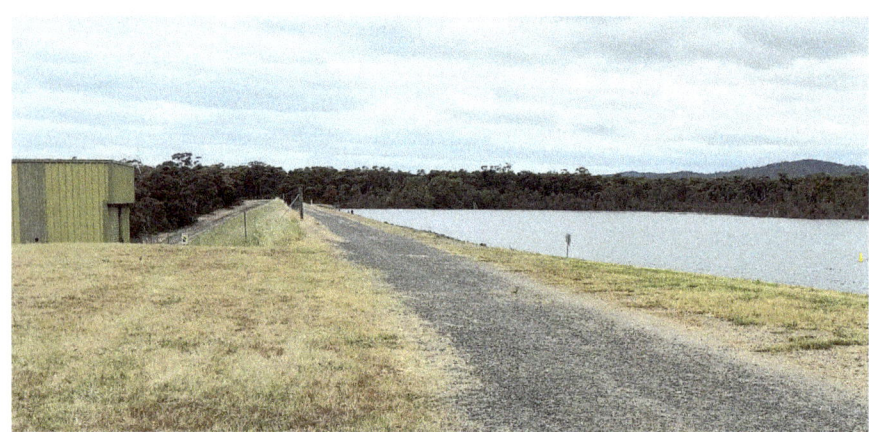

to Specimen Hill and Sparrowhawk. The sites of the "drop" were inspected, and it was observed that it would be quite possible to utilise them for motive power. The principal "drop" will be situated close to the Marong road, at a short distance from Kangaroo Flat. Particular attention was paid to the site at the end of the race at Sparrowhawk Hill, where it is intended to construct a pipehead reservoir for the purpose of increasing the supply to the mains in Sandhurst and Eaglehawk, and thus provide an increased supply of water for domestic purposes. This step has been taken on account of the purity of the water supplied to the Coliban channel from the Malmsbury Reservoir.

It is anticipated that when this work has been completed an abundant supply of water will be provided for domestic purposes during the summer season. The race will accomplish two objects, as it will not only give an additional supply of water for domestic purposes, but the water will be available for sluicing in gullies lying beneath its course. ... The total length of the aqueduct from the Big Hill Reservoir to Sparrowhawk will be 13.5 miles (22 km), so that the work will be one of no small magnitude'
Bendigo Advertiser, Saturday 3 April 1880, p. 3.

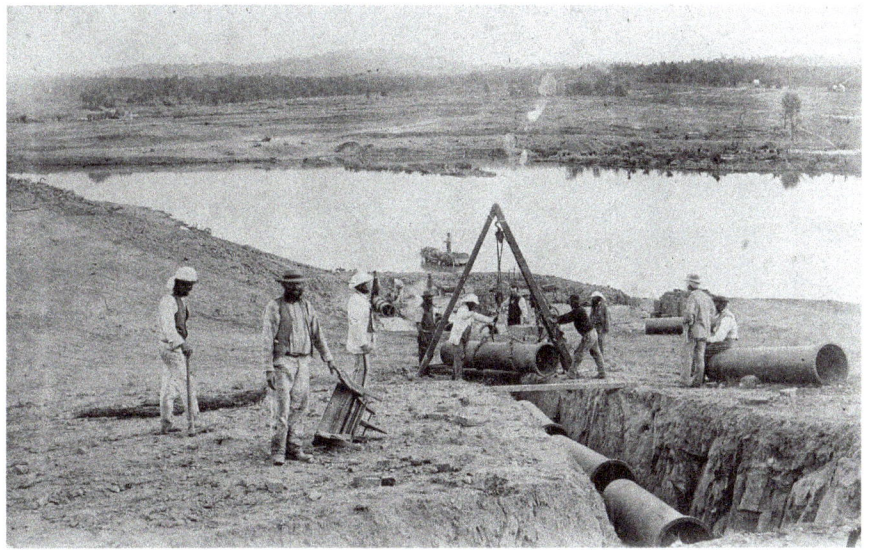
Joseph Brady (behind crane) supervising laying of syphon, 1872.

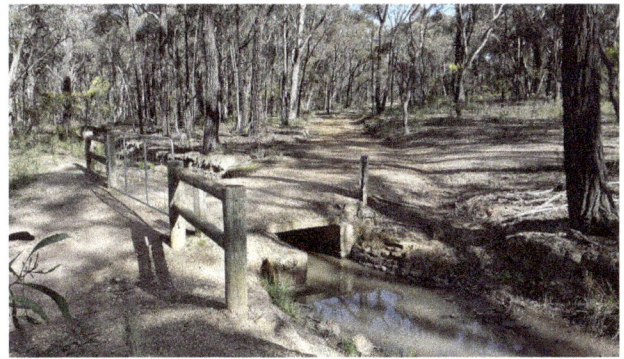
Specimen Hill channel.

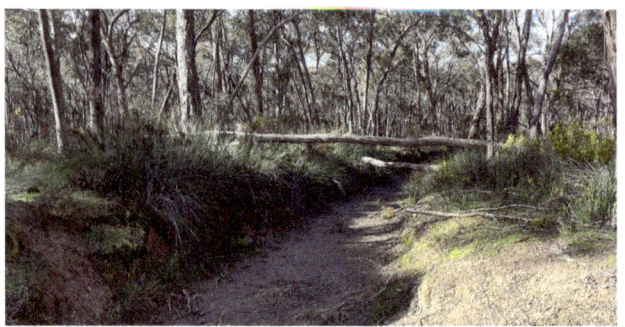
Specimen Hill race.

Continue straight ahead. The track to the right is Thornbill Track. The tracks within the Bendigo Community Parkland have been given new bird names, replacing older names in the process. In a short distance, No. 1 track leads to the left to follow the Specimen Hill race. It makes for a longer walk to follow the race, but it's more attractive, and the whole point of the book has been to follow channels wherever possible!

Along this section there are three watercourses. To the far left, a natural stream bed, next to the track, the Specimen Hill race, and to the right a new catchwater drain which stretches all the way to the Calder Highway, presumably to direct surface water during rain events into the two recreation reservoirs, so augmenting the occasional inflows of Coliban water.

One thing that's apparent is how large the Specimen Hill race is. Either it indicates how much water is sent down the race to Eaglehawk, Marong and Lockwood, or it shows how susceptible the ground is to erosion.

About 2 km from the race bridge, an overshoot makes for a handy bridge to access the northern section of No. 7 Reservoir. Instead of clambering down the rocky chute, turn right and follow the path down to the lakeside track. This might be a good place to take a break.

On your left, the northern bye-wash allows floodwaters to pass down to Bendigo Creek. Near the water's edge there is a long rusting pipe. This is what's left of the pipe which carried water from the Big Hill High Level Reservoir to connect to Bendigo's water supply main.

Retrace your steps over the overshoot and resume walking along the track you'd been on.

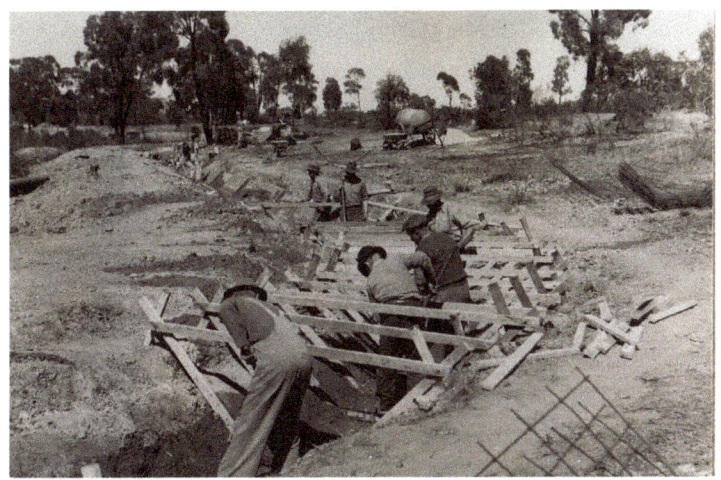

Maintenance works on the Specimen Hill race, October 1946, SR&WSC.

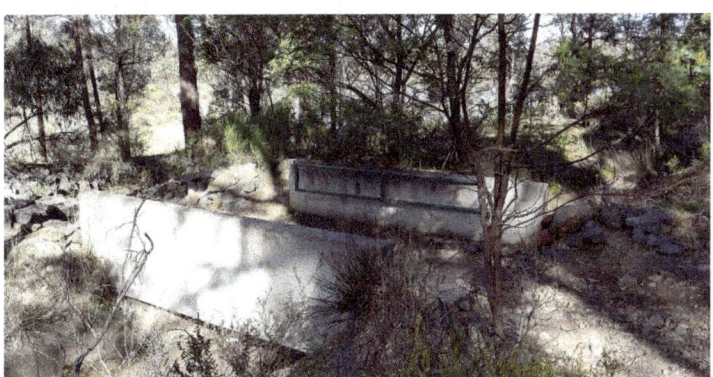

Overshoot leading to No. 7 Reservoir.

At the crossroads, continue straight ahead on Swift Parrot Track (apparently once called High Level Track). Soon you will be following the old High Level pipeline which is underground here. Ahead, the pipe is exposed where it crosses a creek. Nearby there are some valves which once regulated the flow through the pipe.

In 500 metres you will come to the Big Hill High Level Reservoir. This is another decommissioned reservoir, having been replaced by an enormous water tank which these days receives its water by pumps rather than gravity.

A number of historical features are visible here. The high water mark is edged with stones, and the posts and pulleys for raising or lowering the inlet funnel pipe have survived the years.

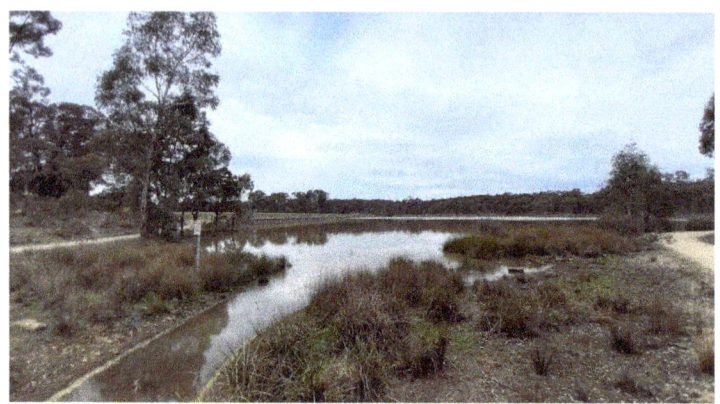

No. 7 Reservoir, north end.

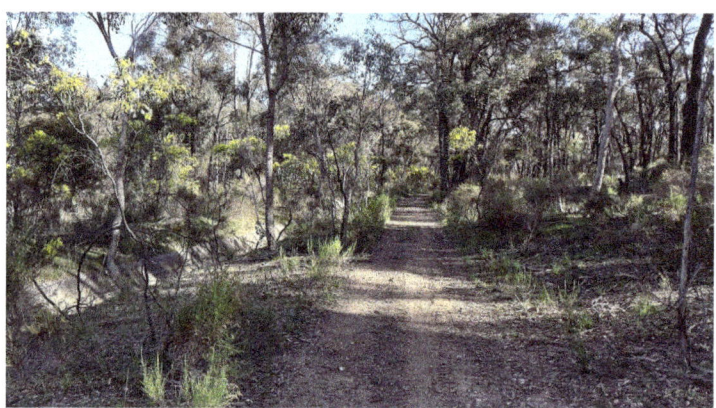

Specimen Hill channel track.

'Another very useful work recently completed is the pipe head reservoir at Big Hill. It was constructed for the purpose of increasing the pressure in Sandhurst, so that the higher portions of the city should be better supplied, and it has proved itself of considerable benefit in that direction. It is situated close to Big Hill [No.7] reservoir, and on a level some 40 feet higher than the settling beds of that reservoir. It is circular in shape, being about 100 feet in diameter, and with sloping sides. ... It is fed direct from the Coliban channel, and the water before entering it is properly purified, and has to pass through very fine brass gauze netting. This reservoir connects directly with the main to Sandhurst and is always kept full'.
Bendigo Advertiser, 31 March 1882, p. 3.

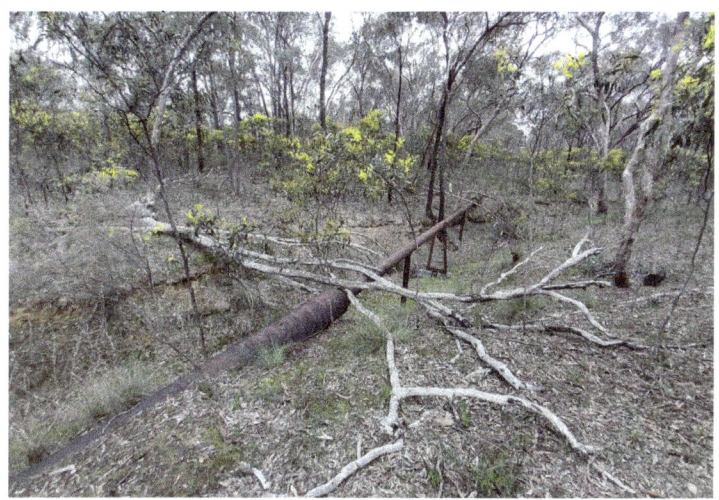
Big Hill High Level Reservoir pipeline.

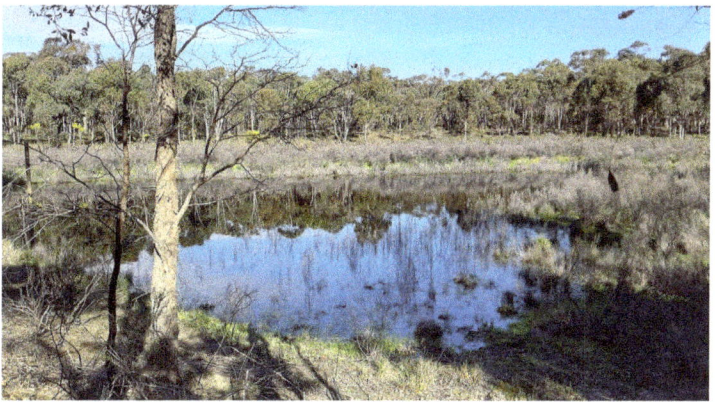
Big Hill High Level Reservoir.

It's difficult to know the fate of this reservoir. Now isolated from an inflow from the High Level channel and not having an extensive catchment, the level of water will probably fluctuate wildly, dependent on the vagaries of yearly rainfall.

Near the reservoir is the Coliban Water pumping station, as well as the water storage tank which, perhaps, has taken over the role of the reservoir in ensuring residents on higher ground in Kangaroo Flat and Big Hill get decent water pressure.

Head around to the outlet of the High Level channel. Follow it along and you will find an old sluice-gate which regulated water inflow, directing it into a gully if necessary.

It's interesting to follow the race for a little while. In a short distance it crosses over a natural creek bed and meets Outlook Track.

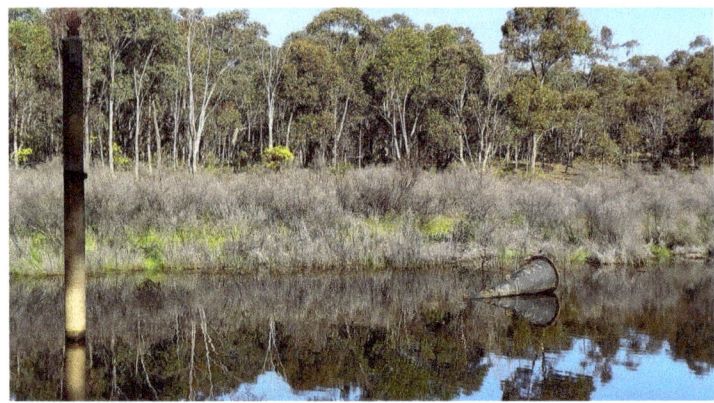

Inlet pipe.

We turn left and within about 300 metres Firetail Track enters Outlook Track from the left. Four signs at each intersection warn us not to dig here or we'll disturb a high pressure gas line.

This is where we turn right to avoid walking on what appears to be a well travelled road. We enter what appears to be a utilities easement, not only carrying a gas pipeline and power line, but also the Coliban water from the storage tank, perhaps to the pumping station near the Calder Highway.

The increasing traffic noise alerts you to your growing proximity to the Calder Highway. Soon, the new catchwater drain is reached. There's no defined path, but if you follow it to your

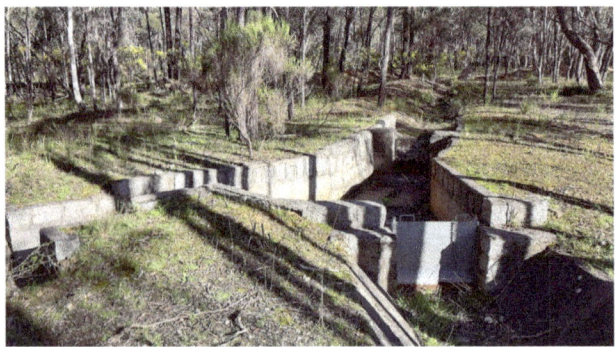

High Level channel sluice gate.

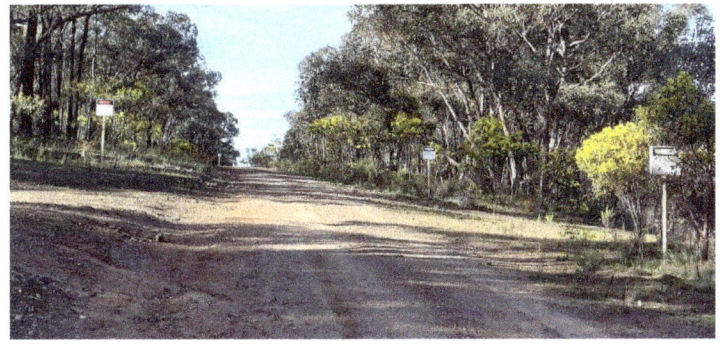

Junction of Firetail and Outlook tracks.

right towards the highway you will see an overshoot and the old Main Channel outlet culvert.

Walkers who have been following the main channel from the east and have crossed the Calder Highway will arrive at this point. The only choice now is to follow the new catchwater drain back towards No. 7 Reservoir, there being no walking track along the old Main Channel.

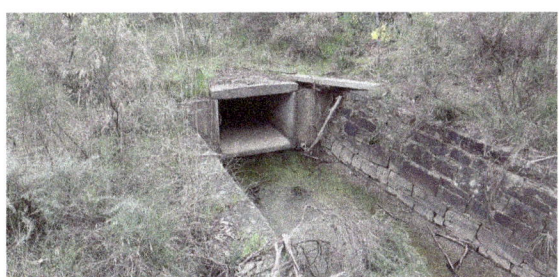

Culvert outlet, Calder Highway.

In 500 metres Outlook Track is met again. Turn right over the bridge. To your right is the Coliban Water Big Hill Urban Supply Station. Oddly, the sign prohibiting access to the facility is on the track access gate rather than on the facility fence itself.

Once over the bridge, turn and walk along the channel. The path is indistinct at the beginning. Within metres you'll reach a point where a photographer stood to capture a visit by inspectors from the SR&WSC in 1946 (see photo page 203).

A little further along the Main Channel there's a very handsome stormwater runoff.

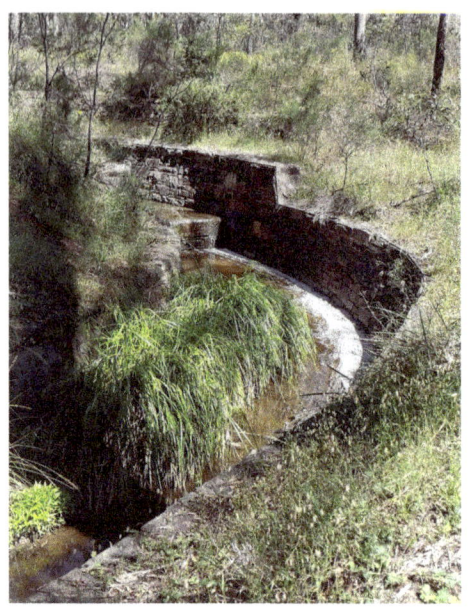

Ahead are the original sluice-gates that regulate the flow of water, either straight ahead into the No. 7 Reservoir or sideways to Crusoe Reservoir.

'The Melbourne road is crossed at 41½ miles [66.79 km] by a culvert, and the Big Hill reservoir [No. 7 Reservoir] is reached at 42½ miles [68.4 km], where by means of sluice-gates the water can be sent direct into it, or at will, into the Crusoe race. The difference of level between these two races at this point is about 40 feet. This is overcome by a step drop similar to that described at the railway crossing. From the foot of this drop to where the channel enters the Crusoe Gully Reservoir, it is about a mile in length.'
Bendigo Advertiser, Tuesday 20 November 1877, p. 3.

Main Channel near Calder Highway.

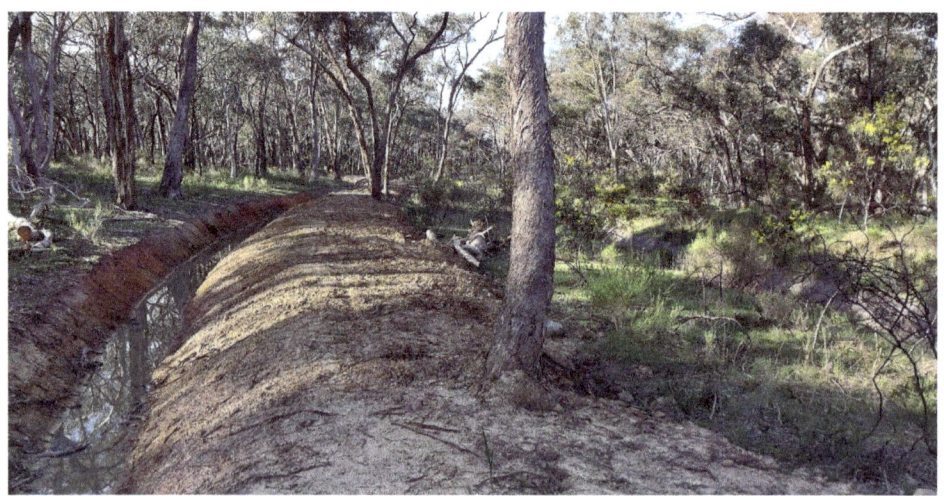

Recently excavated catchwater drain, No. 7 Reservoir.

'The scholars attending the Presbyterian Sunday School at Kangaroo Flat held their annual picnic at the Big Hill reservoir, and had a pleasant outing. Out-door games and pastimes were indulged in. A plentiful supply of cakes, buns, sandwiches, etc., were distributed to the children at intervals. The success of the picnic was greatly due to the untiring efforts of the officers and teachers.
Bendigo Advertiser, Saturday 29 March 1902, p. 5.

If continuing along the channel past the sluice-gates, at least at this stage, there are no signs prohibiting entry. However, if you go far enough and reach the wire fence blocking access to the lakeside

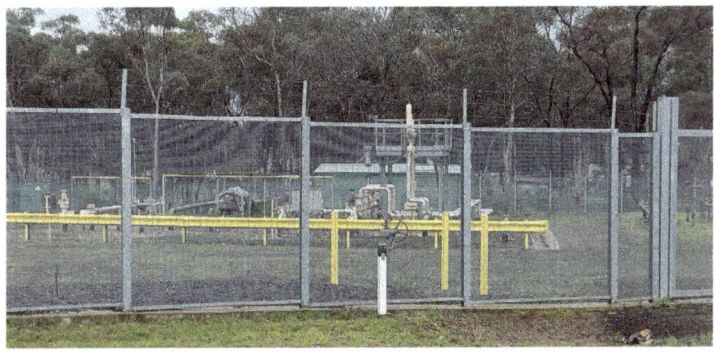

Coliban Water Big Hill Urban Supply Station.

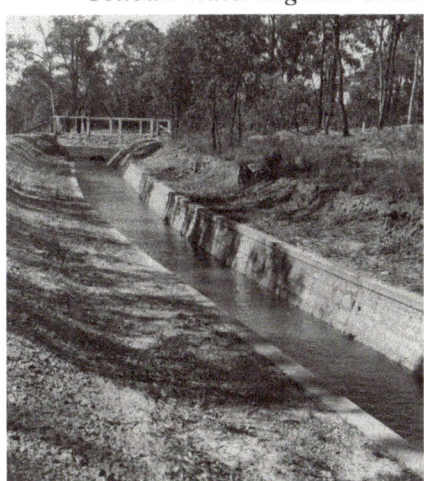
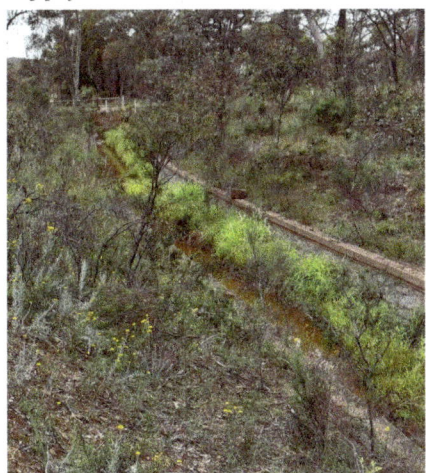

Bridge near Big Hill Urban Supply Station, 1946, SR&WSC.
Right: Present day view of this location.

track, you will discover that, by the Do Not Enter sign hanging on the fence (facing away from you), you shouldn't be there. So at the moment it's best to turn around at the sluice-gates and head back the way you came, turning left at the first side drain you come to. There's a faint vehicle track here which leads to an access track which is the extension of Granter Street.

Turn left here and this will take you back to the car park. On the way you will cross over the Main Channel on its way to Crusoe Reservoir. In 1946, the SR&WSC inspectors parked their car here while they had a look at the channel infrastructure.

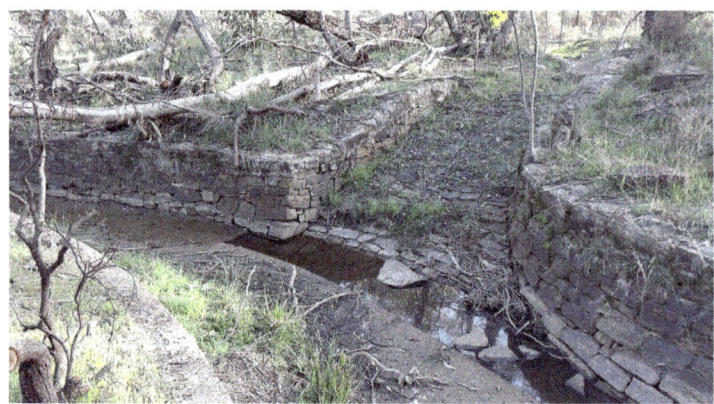

Channel near No. 7 Reservoir.

The car park and facilities are just ahead of you. However, if you didn't get a chance to see it earlier, it's worth having a look at the clear water receiving tank. It's close to the southern edge of the embankment. There's some doubt about its purpose. An interpretive sign nearby has this to say: 'The function of the round brick-lined basin remains a mystery. It was fed via an underground pipe from the adjacent channel and held 554,000 litres of water. The Basin has been dated to have been built in 1876, around the same time as the Coliban Channel. One theory is that it was built as a third settling pond. Or as a header tank to flush out the lime settling ponds. Another theory is that it was used as a header tank to provide large quantities of water quickly for fire fighting purposes.'

So, that's the linear story of the Coliban Main Channel. However, for you long distance walkers, there's still the problem of getting home. Perhaps you started out from Melbourne and came up by train to Malmsbury train station to start your long trek there. Or perhaps you've parked your car at the station and you need to catch a train back to it. So this last walk is for you.

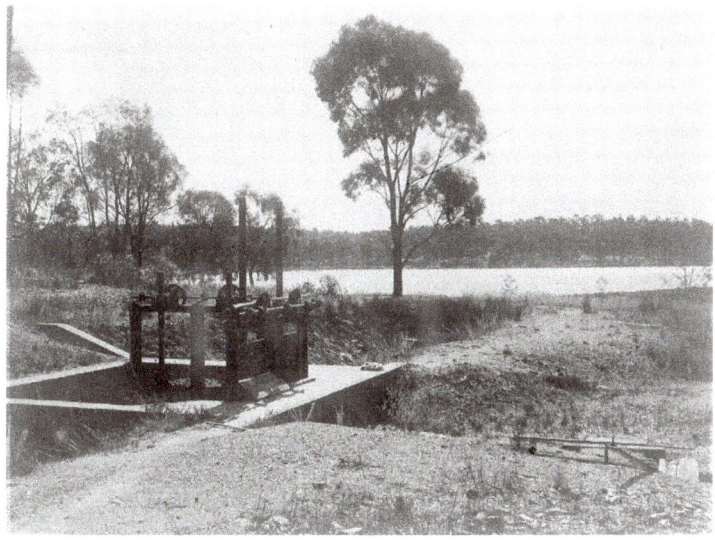

Sluice-gates at No. 7 Reservoir, Cameron, T.W. 1938.
Below: Present day view.

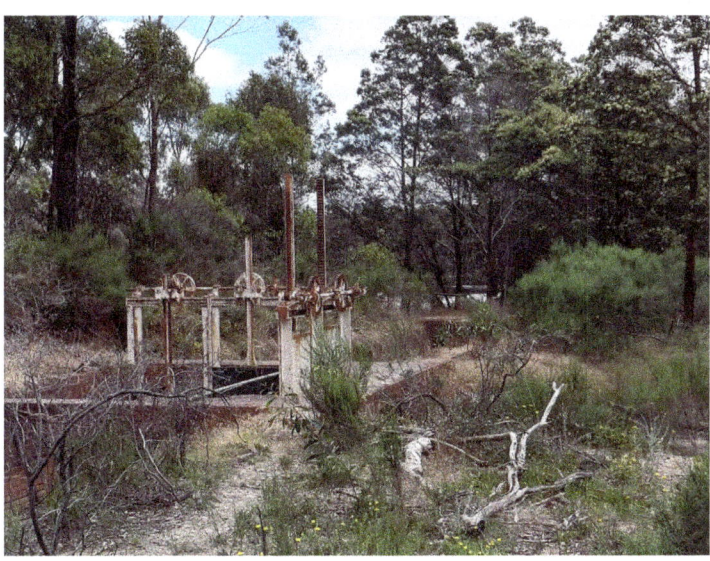

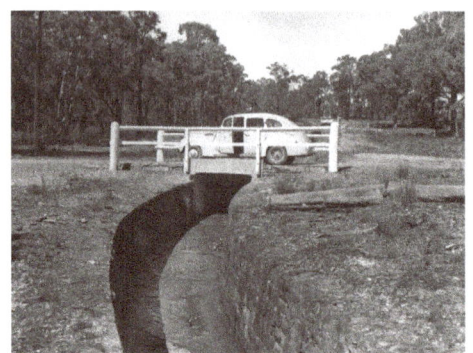 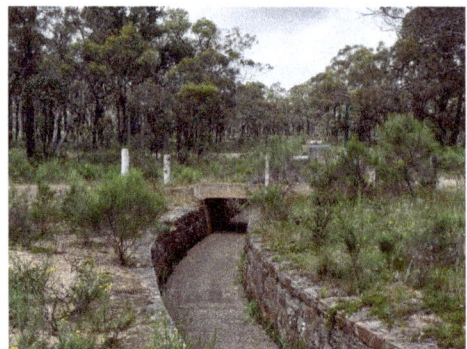

Channel at No. 7 Reservoir, 1946, SR&WSC. Right: Present day view.

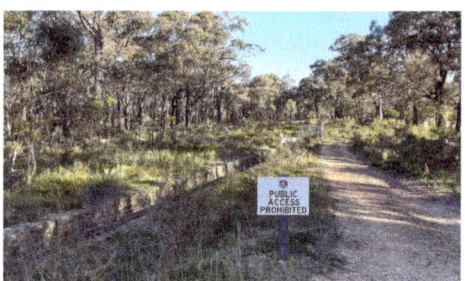

Restricted access here.

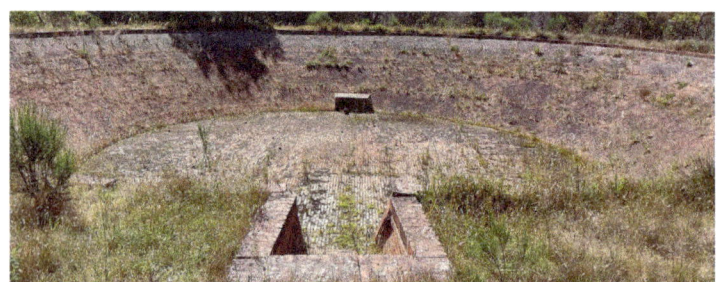

Clear water receiving tank, No.7 Reservoir.

No. 7 Reservoir to Kangaroo Flat Railway Station

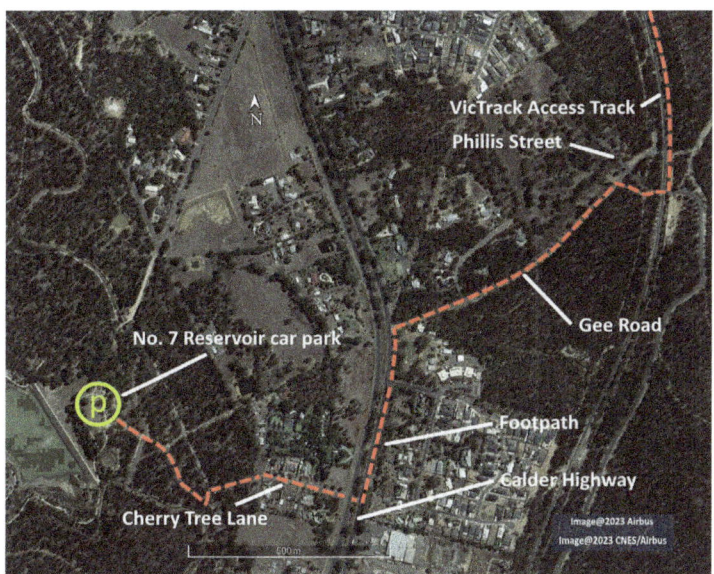

Starting from the shelter at No. 7 reservoir, head south and then turn left at the roundabout on to the track heading east. Walk between the posts next to the gate (see below).

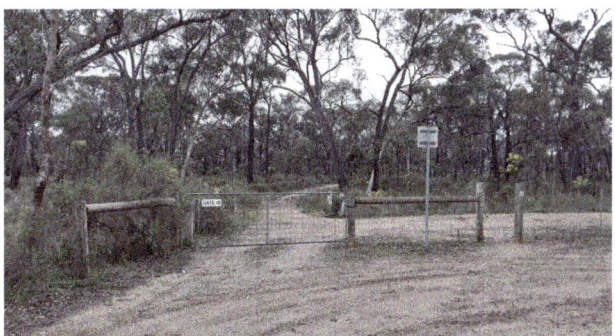

Follow the track for 300 metres and then turn hard left at the next track intersection. Almost immediately, after some logs lying by the track, a trail leads off through the forest on your right.

In about 130 metres there is a fence opening which allows an exit to Cherry Tree Lane, a short street which leads to the Calder Highway.

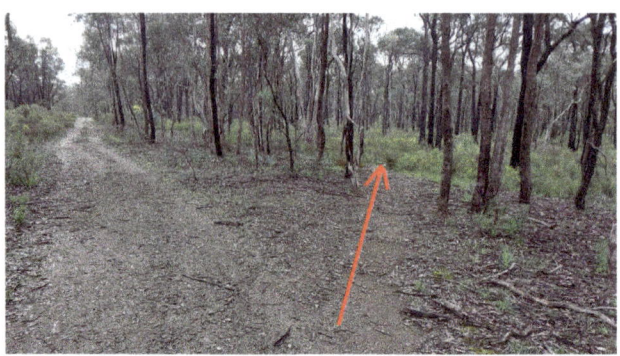

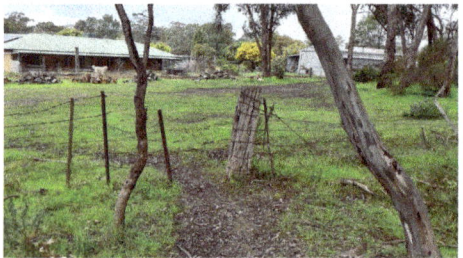
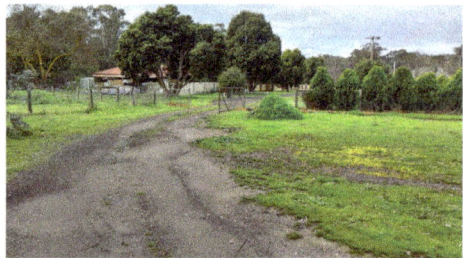

Foot track leading to Cherry Tree Lane.

At the Calder Highway there's no other option but to cross it. The median strip comes in handy. On the other side, a shared bike track/footpath leads to Gee Road. Turn right. After about 200 metres it turns into a delightful rural lane with bushland on the right-hand side.

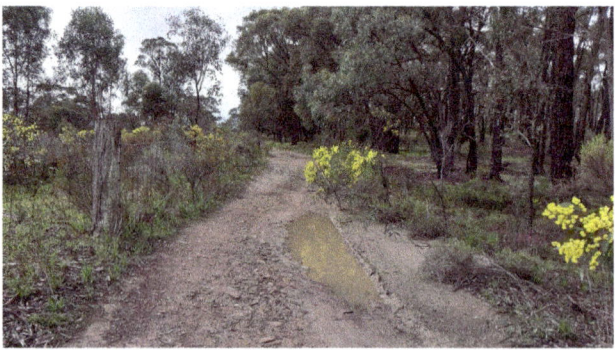

Gee Road.

Just short of Phillis Street there's a shortcut on your right which leads to the railway bridge. Once over the bridge, turn left onto the VicTrack railway access track and you can follow that all the way to the Kangaroo Flat railway station.

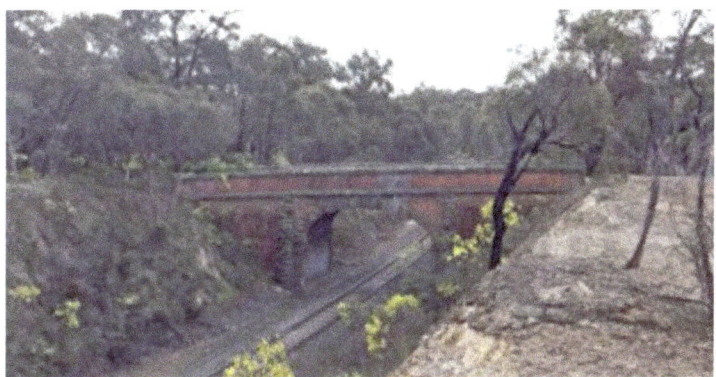

Phillis Street railway bridge.

Epilogue

A very long time ago, when I was young, East Thornbury, a Melbourne suburb, was semi-rural. Hard to believe now. It had farms and paddocks, wild ducks nesting in reed beds and green bell frogs. It also had a channel. It wasn't a grand one. It rose from Darebin Creek near Murray Road, East Preston (which hadn't long been extended through to the Heidelberg side of Darebin Creek). The channel meandered through the paddocks, passed by close to my childhood home, then did a sudden turn to the east to empty back into the lower Darebin Creek.

There was something magical about it to me as a young child. I can still see it in my mind's eye today. Choked with reeds and barely flowing in those days, it invited exploration in a way that the wild, blackberry-infested Darebin Creek didn't.

When I moved to Central Victoria, once again I found myself within a short walk of a channel, but this was the Coliban Main Channel which seemed to go on forever.

We live in a risk averse society these days. Anything that could conceivably hurt someone one day is in danger of being locked away behind high chain link fences, because that's the way insurance companies want it.

Unlike that old East Thornbury irrigation channel, now reduced to an underground stormwater drain, the Coliban main channel still survives, unkempt and undeveloped. So, while we're still able to, it's worth exploring. Long may it rain!

Glossary

Equivalent present day terms are shown in brackets.

abutment: the substructure at the ends of a flume which provide vertical and lateral support for the span.

berm: flat strip of land, raised bank or terrace bordering a channel.

bye-wash (spillway): now generally known as a spillway, it funnels excess water away from the main reservoir embankment to safeguard its structural integrity.

catchwater drain (catch drain): a channel excavated above the main channel and designed to redirect surface waters either to the main channel or, more usually, to a culvert under the main channel, allowing the discharge of those waters into a natural watercourse.

channel: a natural or constructed open conduit with well-defined sides (banks). Also known as an aqueduct or race.

chute: a short open channel that conveys water down a steep slope.

control valve: a valve used in a conduit that can be partly opened to regulate flow or pressure.

copings or cope-stones: capping stones.

culvert: a short tunnel conveying water under roads or railway embankments. When it has a rectangular section it is termed a box culvert.

floodway: a large culvert allowing the passage of floodwaters.

horseshoe breakwater (energy dissipater): a structure designed to absorb the excess kinetic energy of rapidly flowing water.

drop (drop structure, gradient check): an open channel structure specifically designed to provide a rapid change of water level to protect the channel from scouring by the overly fast flow of water. Usually it will have a floor of stone or concrete.

flume, fluming: a stone, brick, wood or iron 'bridge' designed to carry water across a depression, gully or ravine.

level crossing: a point on the channel where the channel bottom is not far above the watercourse it is crossing.

overshoot (abbr. shoot) or shute: a structure of varying shape and material which straddles the channel. It allows water from the high ground above the channel to flow over to the lower ground without entering the channel.

puddle: worked clay which is impervious to water.

stormwater runoff: fortified entry point for surface water to enter the main channel. Usually lined with stone or brick.

sluice-gate, side sluice (flood-gate, flood escape): a barrier that can be lowered to regulate the flow of water. A barrier in the side of the channel that can be raised to allow water to flow out into a natural watercourse below the channel.

step drop (cascade): a succession of small steps in a watercourse or channel that is intermediate in fall between rapids and a waterfall.

syphon (siphon): a pipe, usually buried, which conveys water across a gully to a point of lower elevation, enabling water to flow between those two points.

trash grate: infrastructure which allows the removal of heavy litter from the channel.

waste weir (stormwater overpour): a reinforced section of the channel bank designed to direct overflowing flood waters away while preventing bank erosion.

weir (low level weir): a structure or wall built aross a channel, drain or watercourse to raise the water level to allow diversion or measurement of discharge rate.

Refer: 'Glossary of Terms Used in the Stormwater Industry', Stormwater Australia, 2009

www.ingramcontent.com/pod-product-compliance
Lightning Source LLC
Chambersburg PA
CBHW062033290426
44109CB00026B/2619